Lap Band Weight Loss Diet

Weight Loss Surgery Cookbook, Bariatric Cookbook

Richard P. Russel

Lap Band Weight Loss Diet: Weight Loss Surgery Cookbook, Bariatric Cookbook

This book was self-published with the amazing help of <u>Self-Publishing Made Easy Now!</u> [1] . You can grab a free copy of the checklist that started my journey here: <u>FREE Self-Publishing Checklist</u> [2] .

[1] https://selfpublishingmadeeasynow.com/xpjv
[2] https://selfpublishingmadeeasynow.com/free_checklist

Table of Contents

Book 1 - Weight Loss Surgery Cookbook

Perfect Bariatric-Friendly Recovery Diet After Gastric Bypass (Lifelong Eating, Puree, Maintain Weight Loss, Skinny)

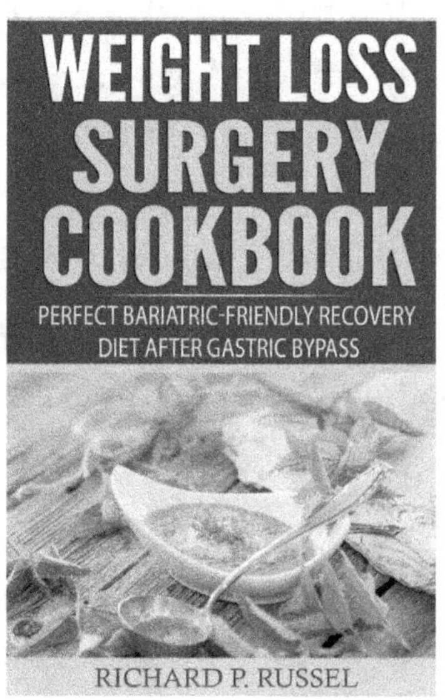

1 - Introduction

I want to thank you and congratulate you for buying this book.

This book contains proven steps and strategies on how to understand what to do after undergoing gastric bypass surgery. This contains information that will help you in coping with the changes and in learning what to do as the healing process progresses.

This book has a wide variety of recipes that are suited for every stage of the healing process. This teaches you about meals and dishes that you can come up with in order to maintain weight loss and make sure that you will benefit from the process for a long time.

Thanks again for buying this book, I hope you enjoy it!

2 - An Overview about the Gastric Bypass Surgery

Known as the most invasive weight loss procedure, the gastric bypass surgery offers the most efficient technique to losing weight. This is ideal for people who are obese or overweight with above 40 Body Mass Index or BMI. Patients at this rate are tagged as morbidly obese.

They are likely suffering from weight-related health problems, which include sleep apnea, high blood pressure, and type 2 diabetes. If you are at this point in your life, the surgery will not only help you lose weight to look good and feel better about yourself but most importantly, it can improve your health and the quality or your life.

The procedure creates a new stomach pouch that is the same size as an egg or a golf ball. A smaller pouch will limit the amount of food that you can take. With a smaller stomach, you will feel less hungry and would only crave to eat smaller portions. The surgery attaches a part of the small intestine to the new pouch.

This allows food to bypass most of the small intestine. As a result, the body absorbs a limited amount of nutrients and calories. This is the main cause of the weight loss – the food that you eat is absorbed less readily by the body.

Before the surgery, your medical team will ask you to follow a pre-operative diet to reduce the size of your liver. The operation is life-changing. Once done, you will modify your dietary habits to last a lifetime. Your surgeon will advise you to follow a staged gastric bypass diet. You will begin with a full liquid diet and it will gradually progress until you are on a normal diet.

Through the dietary changes, your medical team will guide you and tell you when it is safe to progress. They will also give you supplements and medications to make the process of healing faster. You will also be given vitamins, supplements, and minerals that you can take for the rest of your life.

It is important to remember that since your body will be taking in fewer calories, you have to choose the right food to eat in order to maintain a healthy and balanced diet.

3 - The Healing Process

It will take up to 8 weeks for your pouch to completely heal. Planning your meals is important. Your goal is not only to lose weight but also to keep your lean body mass or muscles. Each meal must contain high amounts of protein and low amounts of sugar and fat.

After the operation, your pouch is like that of a baby and it can only absorb liquid and pureed items during the first weeks. This is the purpose of this book – so that you would know what to eat depending on what level you are in.

As you progress in the diet, you can still eat the food items from the previous stages. Whenever you find it hard to tolerate a food item, eliminate it first from your diet for a couple of weeks before reintroducing it to your daily diet.

The Mindful Eating Technique

You will apply this eating technique before and after the surgery. Be always mindful not only of what you eat but how you do it. Consume your food at least 30 minutes or longer, especially in the first weeks following the surgery. Take your time in chewing your food to a liquid consistency. You must also drink slowly.

Do not finish your food if your body already feels full. Put the food away immediately before you get tempted to have another bite.

Helping Yourself Heal Faster

Your dietitian will guide you throughout the process to make it easier for you to make the right food choices. He/she will address your needs after your pouch has thoroughly healed and you are on the last stage of the diet by giving you the nutritional guidelines that you need to follow for the rest of your life.

Here are some important points that you need to remember

The procedure will create an impact and big changes in your life. The struggle is not only physical but also emotional and mental. There are times when you will feel fat even though you are not. It is normal to feel anxious, especially when you hear people's comments about the changes in you.

Always remember that you are not alone in the journey. Join post-operative support groups because they will help a lot in making you more emotionally stable. You must also never lose communication with your medical team. Tell them about your progress and ask for their advice whenever you are going through something that you don't understand.

Help keep the weight off, build and maintain your muscle mass by exercising. Get the approval of your clinician before participating in resistance and cardiovascular training. If you are still not allowed to perform these exercises, opt for simple exercises like walking.

Losing weight is like a plight to a staircase. There are times when it will slow down and times when you will experience plateaus. If the plateau happens for more than 2 weeks, track your exercise and record what you eat. You can adjust your diet and exercise and see if there is any improvement.

If it lasts for more than 4 weeks, get the help of your dietitian and show to him/her your diet and exercise records. Never compare yourself to others who have undergone the same process. Different people will lose weight at different rates.

Here are some of the nutrition considerations following your gastric bypass operation

Maintain a daily fluid intake of 64 ounces or more, depending on your dietary requirement. This will keep your body hydrated by replacing the lost fluids as you lose weight. Separate the fluids from your meals by half an hour. Do not drink while eating a regular meal because the fluids will fill your pouch faster.

Know your daily protein requirement and always meet your protein goals. This helps in the healing process and in preserving your body muscles.

Always follow the mindful eating process. Take tiny bites, eat slowly and eat small frequent meals.

There are instances when you will experience the Dumping syndrome. This happens after eating high sugary and high-fat foods. The symptoms are similar to flu, such as sweating, nausea, diarrhea, and vomiting. These symptoms typically last for 30 minutes. You can avoid experiencing these symptoms by eating foods with around 3 to 5 grams of fat and 14 grams of sugar or less per serving.

There are certain patients who experience hair loss after the surgery. Lack of vitamins and proteins in the diet usually cause this problem. This is also how your body reacts to rapid weight loss. Tell your dietitian if you are experiencing hair loss so that he/she can adjust your vitamins and protein intake. This problem is temporary and the hair grows back normally again after 3 to 6 months.

It is also common to experience a honeymoon period after the operation. It is normal to lack appetite but never make it an excuse to skip meals. You need to meet your daily nutritional requirement and always follow the diet plan of 4 to 6 small meals per day.

Your food preferences may vary as you develop changes in taste.

Many patients experience lactose intolerance after the surgery characterized by diarrhea, cramping, bloating or gas. These are symptoms that you have developed lactose intolerance from the sugar found in milk. Tell your dietitian so that he/she can design a lactose-free diet. This issue will naturally resolve in 3 to 6 months.

Keep records of your meals each day. These logs will help you keep track of the time and frequency of your meals, and what you have eaten.

You need to go to your doctor whenever it is time for a follow-up and check-up. Your labs have to be tested periodically to check if you are not lacking nutrients and vitamins. After the surgery, the most common deficiencies that you are at risk of include Vitamin D, B12, Iron, and Folate.

4 - Dietary Stages after Undergoing Gastric Bypass Surgery

Life after the operation won't be a breeze. You are in a healing process and it will only succeed with your full cooperation. Always remember that your diet will change drastically. You will eventually have the chance to grab a bite or two of your favorite dish, but before that day comes, you need to religiously follow what's allowed to eat depending on the healing phase that you are in.

This book contains a detailed guide about the dietary stages following your gastric bypass surgery.

5 - The First Period: The Fluid Phase

This period refers to the first two weeks following the surgery. The diet aims to help the surgical wounds and the sutures between the small intestines and stomach heal at a faster rate. At this point, you cannot eat too fast or too heavy.

The sutures are still fragile. Eating foods that are unsuitable for this period of the healing process can lead to rupture of the sutures, which can cause the leakage of the contents of your intestines into the abdominal cavity.

Listen to your body. Stop eating once you feel any pain and discomfort even if you feel like you are still not full. This is the body's signal that it has already eaten enough.

Day 1

After the surgery, you are only allowed to consume 1 ounce of water every hour. You will drink from a medicine cup. You have to sip the water in a slow manner. Stop drinking if it makes you feel sick. You will be given swabs to moisten your dry mouth, which is typical to happen at this point.

Day 2

You are still in the hospital at this point. You will be allowed to consume clear liquids one day after the surgery. You can consume 3 ounces of bouillon and/or sugar-free gelatin thrice a day. You can sip plain water or a flat diet ginger ale in between your meals. Your goal is to sip up to 4 ounces of fluid per hour in between your meals.

Aside from nutrition, it is important that you walk as much as you can, not unless your doctor advises you against it. Have a family member or a nurse assist you all the time to ensure your safety.

Day 3 Onwards

After Day 2, you will follow a high-protein full liquid diet. You will do this for 2 weeks. Your goal is to take in at least 64 ounces of fluids per day. Your protein intake per day must be 50 to 60 grams for women and 60 to 70 grams for men and women who are taller than 5'8". Aim for 400 to 600 kilocalorie per day.

You have to eat and sip in a slow manner. Stop at once when your body feels sick or it tells you that it is full. Make sure that you can suck your drinks using a straw and they do not contain lumps and bits. Never gulp your drinks or else you might feel nauseated or even vomit. To avoid dehydration, you must consume at least 2.5 liters per day, most of which are nutritious liquids.

Here are some samples of the healthy liquids and the required amount that you can take at this stage:

- 1 to 2 small glasses of unsweetened fruit juice

- Slimfast

- 1 to 2 tablespoons of skimmed milk for every 200 ml of water. You can also use semi-skimmed milk fortified with skimmed milk powder

- Tinned or homemade smooth soup fortified with up to 2 tablespoons of skimmed milk powder.

- Supplements, which include Complan and Build-Up, which are suitable for diabetics

- Homemade smoothies

You can take coffee, water, tea or squash, but take them in

addition to and not in replacement of any healthy liquids in the list above.

A typical meal plan within this period includes 200 ml of fruit juice for breakfast, 200 ml of homemade smoothie in mid-morning, 200 ml of Slimfast for lunch, Build-Up or Complan or 200 ml dilution of skimmed milk in mid-afternoon, 200 ml of Complan or Build-Up for Dinner and 200 ml of fortified soup for a late-night snack. You can take other liquids in between.

You have to practice listening to what your stomach is telling you. Take your time in eating or in this case, in sipping your meals. You can allow up to 30 minutes for each meal. Listen to your stomach and stop eating when it is full.

This comes with the feeling of pressure at the back of the sternum and under the ribcage. You may also feel nauseous, especially during the first week, pain in the stomach region and on the upper part of thorax or shoulder.

It is important that you do not overfill your pouch. This will make the surgery useless. Eating more than what's required will stretch the pouch, which can lead to complications. To be safe, make sure that you are always mindful of what and you are not eating. If you don't feel an empty stomach, set a reminder so that you won't forget to eat on schedule.

- Here is the food that you have to avoid at this stage:

- Fruits and veggies that are tough and raw

- Rice

- Solid food that is not pureed

- Yogurt with big chunks of fruits

- Peas

- Pasta and noodles

- Corn

- Candies and sweets

- Red meat

- Ice cream

- Chunky peanut butter

- Bread

Here is the food that you can gradually incorporate into your diet. Try these one at a time. If you don't feel good about them, drop them from the list and put them back after several days. If your stomach finds it hard to tolerate pureed food, go back to taking clear liquids.

Pureed vegetables, such as green beans, carrots, cauliflower, beetroot, and broccoli.

Vegetable juice and tomato juice

Pureed low-fat casserole or stew with soft vegetables

Pureed apple or peaches

Mashed banana

Minced pork or turkey

Pureed salmon, tuna, white fish or herring

1 egg yolk and egg white

Pureed soups and cream soups

Pudding and yogurt with low-sugar content

Pureed lean turkey or chicken

6 - Liquid Consumption

Make sure that you drink more than 1.2 liters of liquid per day. Drink more, especially when your urine begins to develop a foul smell and when it becomes dark and cloudy. The color of your urine has to be pale yellow. Sip the liquids slowly and take them separately from your meals.

You can take them 30 mins before and after a meal. It is not advisable to drink using a straw. You will swallow more air when you use a straw, which can lead to belching that will cause pain in the upper thorax and shoulder.

Avoid carbonated drinks and anything that contains too much sugar. Anything that has more than 20 grams of sugar for every 240 ml may cause dumping syndrome, which symptoms include spasmodic pain, dizziness, nausea, and flushing. It is important that you keep a bottle of water with you all the time. This way, it won't be difficult to remember to drink often in a slow manner to avoid dehydration.

Here's a list of the allowed drinks in this phase:

- Water

- Ice cubes

- Non-carbonated flavored water

- Juices diluted in water

- Protein-loaded fruit drinks

- Decaffeinated tea

- Decaffeinated coffee (drink it when warm and not hot)

- Sugar-free popsicles

- Power Aid Zero

- Fat-free and low sodium broth

Here are the drinks that you ought to avoid:

- Carbonated drinks

- Soft drinks

- Drinks with sweet sugar

- Sports drinks

Preparing Your Own Smoothies

Your smoothies must have a watery consistency. Aside from the fruits, each preparation must contain flavorings, liquid, and protein. You can use any fruits – fresh, conserved or frozen. If you want the drink to be thicker, use frozen fruits or add ice cubes when using fresh fruits.

For the liquid, you can choose from soymilk, milk, and protein drink. If you don't like to add the latter, you can instead put 50 ml of yogurt, cottage or ricotta cheese to the mixture. For flavorings, you can use salt, ginger, parsley, cinnamon, dill, cardamom, parsley, and clove. Experiment on the taste by first adding 1/8 teaspoonful of the flavor. Add more according to taste.

Here are some samples of the smoothie mixtures that you can concoct:

- 25 ml each of milk, tofu, and mashed pineapple, ice cubes, and 1/8 teaspoon of ginger

- 25 ml each of cottage cheese and pureed frozen berry mix, 1/8 teaspoon of crushed nutmeg, and 50 ml of protein drink

- 25 ml each of vanilla-flavored yogurt and pureed frozen peaches, 1/8 teaspoon of cinnamon, and 50 ml of protein drink

7 - Allowed Vitamins and Medicines

- Omeprazole tablets. You will be given a prescription for the tablets that you will take for 4 weeks.

- Multivitamin. Start taking 1 tablet two times a day from the second postoperative week.

- Vitamin B12 replacement therapy with injections. This will be administered once every 3 months. The first shot will be given before getting discharged from the hospital.

- Clexane injection once daily for 10 days.

Physical Activity

Make sure that you don't lift more than 6 kilos of weight. Move as much as you can as soon as possible after undergoing the procedure. Your body easily gets tired due to the decreased daily consumption of calories. Rest if you must but go walking whenever you can. You can make the trek more difficult to challenge yourself, such as walking on an uneven surface or walking up and down the stairs.

Other Diet Tips for this Phase

You will lose weight because of the dramatic decrease in your caloric intake. This is why it is important to choose products that are sugar-free or labeled as with no sugar added.

- There are times when you will experience dry mouth even after you have consumed the daily fluid requirement. This is a sign of dehydration and that you need to drink more.

- Do not forget to take or inject the prescription medications that you were given upon your release from the hospital.

- Get in touch with your medical team for any pain and other problems that are causing too much inconvenience.

Meeting the Daily Protein Requirement

Here's a detailed list of the food choices at this stage and how much protein and calories they contain per serving.

- 8 ounces of ready to drink Carnation Instant Breakfast with no sugar added contain 13 grams of protein and 150 calories

- 8 ounces of skim milk with Carnation Instant Breakfast with no sugar added contain 13 grams of protein and 150 calories

- 8 ounces of ready to drink Slimfast contain 10 to 20 grams of protein and 220 to 180 calories

- 11 ounces of ready to drink EAS AdvantEdge contain 17 grams of protein and 110 calories

- 8 ounces of Lactaid skim milk contains 8 grams of protein and 80 calories

- 8 ounces of Simple Smart fat-free milk contains 10 grams of protein and 90 calories

- 8 ounces of skim milk contains 8 grams of protein and 90 calories

- 2 egg whites contain 8 grams of protein and 34 calories

- 1/2 cup of scrambled liquid egg substitute contains 12 grams of protein and 60 calories

- 1/4 cup of fat-free ricotta cheese contains 6 to 10 grams of protein and 40 to 80 calories

- 1/2 cup of fat-free or 1 percent of cottage cheese contains 13 to 14 grams of protein and 70 to 80 calories

- 6 to 8 ounces of light yogurt contain 5 to 8 grams of protein and 60 to 120 calories

- Low-fat or fat-free cream soups mixed with 8 ounces of skim milk contain 10 grams of protein and 190 calories

- 1/2 cup of fat-free or sugar-free instant pudding contains 4 to 5 grams of protein and 75 to 100 calories

Sample Meal Plan

Here's a meal plan that will yield 59 grams of protein, 530 calories, and 56 ounces of fluids:

Begin your day by taking your fluids from 7 to 7:30. In this sample, consume 12 ounces of water. From 8 to 9:00 in the morning, consume your first meal, which is 8 ounces of light yogurt. Take your fluids, 12 ounces of crystal light, from 9:30 to 11:30. Consume your 2nd meal, which is Slim Fast, from 12 noon to 1:00. Take your fluids again, 8 ounces of water, from 1:30 to 3:00.

Take your third meal, 1/2 cup of egg beaters, from 3:30 to 4:00. From 4:30 to 6:00, take your fluids, which is 24 ounces of Power Aid Zero. You will consume your 4th meal from 6:30 to 7:30, which is sugar-free Jello pudding. The last meal of the day is 1/2 cup of cottage cheese that should be eaten from 9:00 to 9:30.

As you can see, everything is monitored, including the amount of time that you will spend consuming each meal. Always take it slow, from 30 to 45 minutes. This will make it easier for your pouch to absorb the foods and all the nutrients that they contain.

8 - First Phase Recipes

Always remember that you can only take blended fruits and veggies, and mix with shakes.

Wild Berry Boost

Place the following ingredients in a blender:

- 8 blueberries

- 4 strawberries

- 4 raspberries

- 1/2 cup of ice cubes

- 8 ounces of non-fat milk

- 2 scoops of vanilla flavored protein powder

Process all the ingredients until smooth and free of lumps. Transfer to a glass and serve.

The Hulk

Here are the ingredients needed to make this smoothie:

- 8 ounces of low-fat milk or cold water

- 3 ice cubes

- 1/2 tablespoon of sugar-free pistachio pudding mix

- A few drops of peppermint extract or 1 mint leaf

- 2 scoops of vanilla protein powder

Process all the ingredients in a blender until smooth. You can opt to add a drop or 2 of green food coloring to the mixture.

Pumpkin Pie Shake

Blend the following ingredients until smooth:

- 1 cup of ice cubes

- 1 cup of soy milk or skim milk

- 1/4 cup of pumpkin puree

- 1 scoop of vanilla protein powder

- 1/4 cup of vanilla yogurt

- 1/2 teaspoon of pumpkin pie spice

- 2 tablespoons of Splenda granular

Mocha Proticcino

Here are the needed ingredients to make this mix:

- 8 ounces of skim milk

- 1 tablespoon of decaf instant coffee

- 1 scoop of vanilla or chocolate protein powder

Put all the ingredients in a blender and process until smooth. You can tweak the recipe by adding 1/4 banana. Blend until free of lumps. Another way to tweak this is by adding 2 teaspoons of low-sugar peanut butter.

Cinnamon Roll Protein Shake

Put the following ingredients in a blender and process until smooth and free of lumps:

- 1/4 teaspoon of cinnamon

- 1 scoop of vanilla protein powder

- 3 ice cubes

- 1 tablespoon of sugar-free instant vanilla pudding

- 8 ounces of low-fat milk or water

- A dash or two of butter-flavored extract or sprinkles

- 1/4 teaspoon of vanilla extract

- 1 packet of Splenda

Apple Cinnamon

Blend all the ingredients in a blender until smooth:

- 1 teaspoon of cinnamon

- 2 scoops of vanilla whey protein powder

- 1 cup of chopped frozen apple

- 1 1/2 cups of skim milk or water

High-Protein Pudding

To prepare this, you will need a 4-serving package of the uncooked Jell-O sugar-free instant pudding.

Mix 2 scoops of unflavored protein powder and 2 cups of cold skim milk. Shake to mix well. Prepare the Jell-O sugar-free instant pudding according to package directions. Add the milk and protein powder mixture. Mix thoroughly. Chill and serve.

After two weeks, you will need to see your medical team to assess your progress. It is up to your dietitian whether it is safe for you to progress to the next phase of the diet or not. He/she will base the decision on the findings of your doctor.

9 - The Second Period: Soft and Moist Protein Diet

This period covers the third and fourth week after your surgery. For some, this can last up to 6 weeks. It really depends on how your stomach is recuperating and how your whole system is adjusting to the new scheme of things. At this phase, you will have more options of foods to eat.

This is to prepare your stomach for solid food. Your pouch is gradually recovering but it is still not capable of digesting solid food. The food choices that you have during this phase only require minimal chewing.

Your goal is to take in more than 64 ounces of fluids per day. Your protein intake per day is 50 to 60 grams for women and 60 to 70 grams for men and women who are taller than 5'8". Aim for 550 to 700 kilocalorie per day.

At this stage, it is no longer necessary to puree your foods. Mash your foods to make them chewable and do not swallow large chunks. Introduce food items one at a time to check if you can tolerate them. If not, remove them from the diet and try eating them again after a week.

9 - THE SECOND PERIOD: SOFT AND MOIST PROTEIN DIET

Train yourself to eat 3 to 5 small regular meals a day. Continuous nibbling during the day is not advisable because it reduces weight loss. Eat slowly and chew your food thoroughly.

Eating fast may lead to vomiting and the Dumping syndrome. Initially, the connections between the small intestine and stomach are narrow. By eating slowly, the connections guarantee a smooth movement of the food that passes through them.

Always feel the pressure at the back of your sternum beneath the ribcage. This means that you are full and it can happen even after eating 2 to 3 mouthfuls. Monitor the amount of protein that you take all the time. You can consume protein additives if you are finding it hard to meet the required amount from your regular meals.

Here are the foods that you have to avoid at this stage:

- Red meat

- Tough, dry, and hard meat

- Chunky peanut butter

- Fried egg

- Raw fruits with tough skin

- Hard fruits

- Ice cream

- Chewing gum and other sweets

- White bread

- Soft half-baked bread

- Broccoli stems

- Fresh asparagus

- Fats and sugars

Here are the foods allowed to eat in this phase:

- Fruits and vegetables without seeds and soft-boiled husks

- Soft fresh fruits

- Soft and juicy lean meat

- Low-fat cottage cheese

- Fish

- Eggs

- Soft tofu

- Porridges with milk

- Pretzels

- Soft vegetables and fruits conserved in on juice

- Low-fat yogurt

Liquid Consumption

Sip liquids in the same manner as you did in the previous phase. The required amount of fluid intake per day is 1.2 to 1.5 liters. Do not drink half an hour before eating a regular meal. Your stomach has to be empty when you eat. You are also not allowed to drink while eating.

9 - THE SECOND PERIOD: SOFT AND MOIST PROTEIN DIET

This will fill up your pouch fast, which can lead to experiencing the Dumping syndrome, nausea, abdominal pain, and vomiting. Wait 30 minutes or more after eating a meal before drinking liquids. This aims to avoid fast flushing of the food in your stomach.

Here's a list of the allowed drinks to take in this phase:

- Water

- Non-carbonated flavored water

- Juices diluted in water

- Sugar-free tea

Here are the drinks that you ought to avoid:

- Carbonated drinks

- Soft drinks

- Drinks with sweet sugar

- Sports drinks

Allowed Vitamins and Medicines

- Continue taking Omeprazole tablets and Multivitamin

- Vitamin B12 replacement therapy with injections

- 30 microgram D3-vitamin tablet once per day

- 600-milligram Calcium nitrate tablets twice a day beginning on the 3rd day after the surgery

- 100-milligram of iron preparations once every other day for women in fertile age

Physical Activity

It is important to remain as physically active as possible. You can ride a bike, perform Nordic walking, speed walking, or simply walk at times when you are not in the mood to do more than that. You are not allowed to lift more than 6 kilos of heavy objects. You can go swimming 3 weeks after the operation.

Other Diet Tips for this Phase

- Cut your food to a ground consistency. Add sugar-free and fat-free condiments to keep them moist. You can also cook them in ways that they will retain the moisture, such as roasting, baking, poaching, and steaming.

- Since you will be eating your food slowly, you can keep them warm by placing your plate on a baby food warmer tray.

- After cooking your meal, weigh it using a food scale. Aim for about 3 ounces of protein per meal.

- Avoid chewing gum. If you accidentally swallow it, the gum will block the connection to your pouch.

- If you are always meeting your daily protein goals, you can include half a cup of mashed vegetables or mashed potatoes mixed with skim milk to your daily menu and have it once a day.

- If you are often experiencing constipation, add a fiber

supplement to your fluids.

Meeting the Daily Protein Requirement

Here's a detailed list of the food choices at this stage and how much protein and calories they contain per serving.

Vegetarian protein sources:

- 1/2 cup of scrambled liquid egg substitute contains 12 grams of protein and 60 calories

- 2 tablespoons of hummus contain 8 grams of protein and 100 calories

- 1/2 cup of beans, such as refried, black and kidney beans, contains 8 grams of protein and 103 calories

- 3 ounces of fat-free or low-fat cheese contain 20 grams of protein and 124 calories

- 1 large egg contains 6 grams of protein and 78 calories

- 1/2 cup of fat-free or 1 percent cottage cheese contains 15 grams of protein and 80 calories

- 1/2 cup of lentils contains 9 grams of protein and 115 calories

- 1/2 cup of ground soy crumbles contains 11 grams of protein and 70 calories

- 1/2 cup of tempeh contains 16 grams of protein and 165 calories

- 1/2 cup of tofu contains 20 grams of protein and 183 calories

- 1 vegetable burger patty contains 9 grams of protein and 70 calories

Animal protein sources:

- 2.5 ounces of baby food contains 8 grams of protein and 50 calories

- 3 ounces of ground meat contain 21 to 23 grams of protein and 150 calories

- 1/2 cup of turkey chili contains 8 grams of protein and 92 calories

- 3 ounces of canned chicken breast packed in water contain 16 grams of protein and 80 calories

- 3 ounces of fish, such as sole, halibut, and haddock contain 21 to 23 grams of protein and 90 to 120 calories

- 3 ounces of fatty fish like bluefish and salmon contain 21 to 23 grams of protein and 160 calories

- 3 ounces of tuna packed in water contain 20 to 22 grams of protein and 100 to 110 calories

- 3 ounces of scallops, shrimp, and crabmeat contain 14 to 18 grams of protein and 85 to 90 calories

- 3 ounces of skinless turkey or chicken breast contain 25 grams of protein and 120 to 150 calories

- 3 ounces of imitation seafood contain 10 grams of protein and 87 calories

Sample Meal Plan

Here's a meal plan that will yield 74 grams of protein, 445

calories, and 56 ounces of fluids:

Begin your day by taking your fluids from 7 to 7:30. In this sample, consume 12 ounces of crystal light. From 8 to 9:00 in the morning, consume your first meal, which is half a cup of egg beaters. Take your fluids, 8 ounces of water, from 9:30 to 11:30. Consume your 2nd meal, 3 ounces of tuna salad with fat-free mayonnaise, from 12 to 1:00.

Take your fluids again, 24 ounces of Power Aid Zero, from 1:30 to 3:00. Consume your third meal, 8 ounces of light yogurt, from 3:30 to 4:00. From 4:30 to 6:00, take your fluids, which is 12 ounces of water. You will consume your 4th meal from 6:30 to 7:30, which is 3 ounces of haddock and 1/4 cup of mashed potatoes. Eat your last meal for the day, 4 ounces of Greek yogurt, from 9:00 to 9:30.

Second Phase Sample Recipe

Steamed Fish with Yogurt Dill Sauce

Here are the needed ingredients for this dish:

- 1/2 cup of reduced-sodium and fat-free chicken broth

- 1 scallion, finely chopped

- 2 tablespoons of extra virgin olive oil

- 1 tablespoon of fresh dill

- 1 teaspoon of finely minced fresh basil

- 1 lemon, thinly sliced

- Salt and pepper to taste

- 1 tablespoon of finely chopped fresh chives

- 1/3 cup of plain low-fat yogurt

- 4 sprigs of fresh dill for garnish

Mix the basil, chives, half of the dill, and oil in a bowl. Rub the mixture on all sides of the fish. Season with salt and pepper. In another bowl, mix the sauce by combining the yogurt with the rest of the dill.

Arrange the scallions at the bottom of a deep-rimmed serving dish. Put the fish and top with the lemon slices. Add the broth. Cook in the microwave at a medium temperature setting until the fish is easily flaked using a fork. Garnish with dill and serve the dish with the prepared sauce.

10 - The Third Period: High Protein, Low-Fat, Low-Sugar Diet

This period starts one month after the procedure. At this stage, you are feeling better and it is easier to eat bread and meat. This doesn't mean that you can go back to your old eating habits. The success of your weight loss plans still depend on your commitment to eating healthy food and staying away from sweets and alcohol.

There are times when you will find eating and drinking more difficult than the earlier weeks. This means that the connection of the small intestine and stomach is healing. A scar is forming at the connection site, which makes it narrower and thicker. As a result, the movement of anything that you drink or eat takes a longer time to pass through the connection.

At this phase, you can incorporate more solid and easily chewable foods. When eating solid food items, reduce the number of meals you have to three per day but do not go any less than that. The interval between meals is 4 to 5 hours. Concentrate on your food while eating. Cut your food into small portions and allow 20 to 30 minutes in eating each meal.

You must still pay attention to the pressure at the back of your sternum, which signifies that your pouch is full and that you must stop eating. Do not overeat. If it happens often, your stomach will stretch and will make the whole process useless.

Your goal is to take in more than 64 ounces of fluids per day. Your protein intake per day is 65 to 90 grams. Every meal must have a protein-rich food, and make it a habit to eat them first. You can stop taking protein drinks only if you are certain that you are getting the necessary amount of protein from what you eat.

Introduce one new food per day. Eat food items that are low-fat and healthy and avoid anything that contains easily absorbed carbohydrates and sweets. Aim for 900-1000 kilocalorie per day from here on until the end of the first year after undergoing the procedure.

Here are the foods that you may find hard to tolerate this stage

- Fruits with hard skin and many seeds

- Red meat

- Hard or cartilaginous meat

- Whole milk

- Apple

- Ice cream

- Fruits with tough skin

- Grapes

- Fruit bread

- Noodles

- Condensed milk

- Nuts

- Chili and spicy foods

- Rice

- Potato peels

- Grain bread with pieces of fruits and nuts

- Chewing gum

- Sweets

To achieve the biggest weight loss, limit or avoid the following food items:

- Fast noodle food

- High-fat cream soups

- Meat products and vegetables, fried and covered with breadcrumbs

- Condensed milk

- Chocolate milk

- Fried eggs

- Donuts

- Danish pastries

- Fast foods

- Sweet bread

- Fried salty snacks

- Fruits with added sugar

- Ice cream

- Whole milk

Liquid Consumption

Like in the previous phases, you have to sip your liquids in a slow manner. The required amount of fluid intake per day is 1.2 to 1.5 liters. Do not drink half an hour before and after eating.

Here's a list of the allowed drinks to take in this phase:

Water

- Non-carbonated flavored water

- Juices diluted in water

- Sugar-free tea

Here are the drinks that you ought to avoid:

- Carbonated drinks

- Soft drinks

- Drinks with sweet sugar

- Sports drinks

Allowed Vitamins and Medicines

Continue taking the following items from the previous phase:

- 1 multivitamin tablet twice a day

- Vitamin B12 replacement therapy with injections

- 30 microgram D3-vitamin tablet once per day

- 600-milligram Calcium nitrate tablets twice a day

- 100-milligram of iron preparations once every other day for women in fertile age

Physical Activity

It is now time to develop a regular exercise routine. Make sure that you walk at least an hour and 30 minutes every day. You are no longer restricted to lift weights. You can now perform challenging exercises to burn calories and build muscles.

Sample Meal Plan

Here's a meal plan that will yield 735 calories, 69 grams of protein, 9 grams of fat, and 94 grams of carbohydrates.

Breakfast starts at 8 to 8:30. In this sample, eat 1/2 slice of toasted dry whole wheat bread and 1 scrambled egg. Take your snacks and fluids from 9 to 11:30, which include 8 ounces of flavored water, 8 ounces of tea, decaffeinated coffee, or water.

Eat the following for lunch scheduled from 12 noon to 12:30: 2 saltine crackers, 1 cup of lentil soup, 1/2 canned peach with no syrup and no sugar added, and 2 baby carrots. From 2:30 to 5:30, take your snacks and fluids, such as 8 ounces of zero-calorie beverage, 6 ounces of fat-free light yogurt, and 12 ounces of water.

Dinner comes at 6 to 6:30 and is composed of 1/4 cup of steamed rice sprayed with diet margarine, 3 ounces of baked haddock with lemon, 1/4 cup of strawberries, and 1/4 of steamed broccoli. Take your snacks and fluids from 7 to 10 in the evening, which include 12 ounces of flavored water, 1/2 fat-free ricotta cheese, and 12 ounces of water.

11 - Bariatric-Friendly Breakfast Recipes

Here are the recipes that you can prepare when you are in your last phase of the healing period and for the rest of your life to maintain the weight you've lost and keep your ideal figure.

Breakfast Pancakes with Peanut Butter and Jelly

This recipe contains 10 grams of protein, 1.5 grams of fat, 9 grams of carbohydrates, and 90 calories per serving size of 1 pancake.

The following ingredients will yield 4 servings of this dish:

- 4 egg whites

- 2 tablespoons of powdered peanuts

- 1/2 cup of instant oatmeal

- 1/2 cup of low-fat cottage cheese

- 1 cup of frozen mixed berry blend

Process the following ingredients in a blender: cottage cheese, oatmeal, peanuts, and egg whites. Stop the blender once it looks like a pancake batter. Transfer the mixture to a bowl. Fold in the berry fruit mix and cook the pancakes in a greased skillet.

Pumpkin Pie Oatmeal

This recipe contains 14 grams of protein, 3 grams of fat, 34 grams of carbohydrates, and 205 calories per serving.

Here are the needed ingredients to make a serving of this dish:

- 1/2 cup of 1 percent cottage cheese with no salt added

- 1/2 cup of canned pumpkin

- 30 grams of old-fashioned oats

- 1/8 teaspoon of cinnamon

- 1 teaspoon of Truvia baking blend

- A dash each of ground cloves and ground ginger

Put the oats in a heatproof bowl. Add the pumpkin,

sweetener, and spices. Mix well. Cook in the microwave on a high setting for 90 seconds. Stir in the cottage cheese. Put back in the microwave and cook for 60 seconds. Leave at a room temperature for a couple of minutes before serving.

Yogurt Popsicles

This recipe contains 5 grams of protein, 0.6 gram of fat, 11 grams of carbohydrates, and 75 calories per serving size of 1 popsicle.

Prepare the following ingredients to make 6 popsicles:

- 1/2 cup of skim milk or 1 percent milk

- 1 cup of non-fat and plain Greek yogurt

- 1/2 cup or instant or regular oats

- 1 cup of chopped fruits or mixed berries

Mix milk and yogurt in a bowl until combined. Transfer it into 6 popsicle molds. Divide the berries and oats into each mold. Put in the freezer for a minute. Insert popsicle sticks into the molds. Put back into the freezer until set and firm.

Tuna Sandwiches with Apple

This recipe contains 23 grams of protein, 2.5 grams of fat, 30 grams of carbohydrates, and 250 calories per serving size of 1/3 of the recipe.

Get the following ingredients ready to make 3 sandwiches:

- 3 lettuce leaves, rinsed

- 1 6.5-ounce can of tuna, drained

- 1/2 teaspoon of honey

- 1/4 cup of low-fat vanilla yogurt

- 6 slices of whole wheat bread

- 1 apple, peeled, washed, and cut into small pieces

- 1 teaspoon of mustard

Mix the yogurt, apple, mustard, honey, and tuna in a bowl. Lay 3 bread slices and spread them with half of the mixture. Put a lettuce leaf and the other slice of each bread on top of each sandwich.

High-Protein Cottage Cheese Pancakes

This recipe contains 13 grams of protein, 7 grams of fat, 10 grams of carbohydrates, and 152 calories per serving size of 1 pancake.

Here are the necessary ingredients to make 3 servings of the dish:

- 1/3 cup of all-purpose flour

- 1 cup of low-fat cottage cheese

- 1/2 teaspoon of baking soda

- 1/2 tablespoon of canola oil

- 3 eggs, lightly beaten

Mix the flour and baking soda in a bowl. Put the remaining ingredients in another bowl and mix until combined. Gradually combine the two mixtures. Cook 1/3 of the batter at a time in a greased skillet over medium heat. Top the pancakes with low-calorie syrup before serving.

Protein Loaded Pumpkin-Ricotta Pie

This recipe contains 6 grams of protein, 3.5 grams of fat, 10 grams of carbohydrates, and 105 calories per serving size of 1 slice.

Here are the necessary ingredients to make 12 servings of the dish:

- 2-ounce pack of pecan halves

- 1 cup of nonfat milk

- 2 eggs

- 1 teaspoon each of ground nutmeg and ground cinnamon

- 2 scoops of Whey Protein Isolate (100% unflavored)

- 1/2 teaspoon of salt

- 1/3 cup of Splenda Sugar Blend

- 1 cup of part skim ricotta cheese

- 2 cups of 100 percent pure canned pumpkin puree

with no added salt

Put the ricotta cheese, 1/2 cup of milk, and eggs in a blender. Process until smooth. Put the remaining ingredients and process until blended. Transfer the batter to a greased pie dish. Put the pecans on top. Bake for 45 minutes in a preheated oven at 350 degrees. Transfer to a wire rack and leave for an hour to cool. Slice into 12 and serve.

Hot and Spicy Deviled Eggs

This recipe contains 10 grams of protein, 8.7 grams of fat, 1 gram of carbohydrates, and 131 calories per serving size of 2 deviled eggs.

Prepare the following ingredients to make 3 servings of this dish:

- 1/2 teaspoon of dill

- 6 hard-boiled eggs, peeled

- A dash of paprika and black pepper

- 1/8 teaspoon of salt

- 2 tablespoons of Greek yogurt

- 1/4 teaspoon of spicy mustard

Cut the eggs in half. Scoop out the egg yolks. Put the 3 cooked yolks in a bowl and keep the other 3 in the fridge and use for another recipe. Mix the 3 egg yolks and yogurt. Gradually mash while adding the mustard, dill, and salt. Divide the mixture to fill each half of the egg white. Season with pepper and paprika before serving.

Breakfast Egg-Chilada

This recipe contains 23 grams of protein, 8 grams of fat, 3 grams of carbohydrates, and 171 calories per serving size of 1 egg-chilada.

Here are the needed ingredients to make a serving of this dish:

- 2 tablespoons of salsa

- 1 ounce chicken, tofu, or ground beef

- Salt and black pepper to taste

- 1 egg, plus 1 egg white, beaten

- 1 tablespoon of shredded Mexican blend cheese

- 2 tablespoons of plain and fat-free Greek yogurt

Spread the beaten eggs in a greased skillet over medium heat. Allow to set for 2 minutes before sprinkling with salt and pepper. Flip the eggs and cook the other side for a couple of minutes.

Transfer to a plate. In a bowl, combine the protein of choice, chicken, tofu, or ground beef, and cheese. Turn the mixture into a strip and put on top of the egg pancake. Roll the pancake to wrap the filling. Top with salsa and yogurt before serving.

Egg Muffin

This recipe contains 8 grams of protein, 7 grams of fat, 1 gram of carbohydrates, and 98 calories per serving size of 1 muffin.

The following ingredients will yield 12 servings of this dish:

- 12 slices of turkey bacon, cooked and sliced into

thirds

- 1/2 cup of 1 percent milk

- 6 eggs

- 3/4 cup of shredded low-fat Swiss cheese

- 1/4 teaspoon each of Italian seasoning, salt, and pepper

Grease 12 muffin cups. Put 3 bacon slices in each cup. Set aside 1/4 cup of cheese. Put the remaining ingredients in a bowl and mix well. Scoop out 1/4 of the mixture on top of the bacon slices. Sprinkle cheese on top. Bake for 25 minutes in a preheated oven at 350 degrees.

Berry Breakfast Wrap

This recipe contains 8 grams of protein, 9 grams of fat, 30 grams of carbohydrates, and 233 calories per serving size of 1 tortilla wrap.

You will need the following ingredients to make a serving of this dish:

- 1 tablespoon of low-sugar strawberry jelly

- 3 tablespoons of regular ricotta cheese

- 1 tortilla (whole wheat)

- 1/3 cup of sliced fresh strawberries

Lay the tortilla on a plate. Spread it with cheese and jelly. Add the berries on top. Roll the tortilla to wrap the filling.

Quinoa Bowl with Tofu

This recipe contains 12 grams of protein, 10 grams of fat, 27 grams of carbohydrates, and 232 calories per serving size of 1/6 of the recipe.

To make 6 servings of this dish, you will need the following:

- 2/3 cup of chopped scallions

- 1 15-ounce pack of extra firm tofu, diced

- 1 cup of shredded carrots

- 1 cup of uncooked quinoa

- 1 tablespoon of sesame oil

- 2 tablespoons of soy sauce

- 1/2 cup each of fresh cilantro and toasted slivered almonds

- 1 1/2 cups of chicken broth

For the sauce, you will need:

Juice of 1/2 lime

- 1 teaspoon of grated ginger

- 1 garlic clove, minced

- 2 tablespoons each of rice wine vinegar and Sriracha sauce

- 1/2 tablespoon of brown sugar

- 3 tablespoons of coconut milk

- 2 teaspoons of creamy peanut butter

Rinse the tofu and drain the liquid 30 minutes before cooking. Transfer them to a plate lined with a dish towel. Place another plate on top. This will provide the weight to get rid of the excess liquid.

Leave for half an hour. Put the sesame oil, tofu, and soy sauce in a bowl. Toss to combine. Transfer to a baking sheet and bake for 40 minutes. Toss the ingredients every 10 minutes and continue baking until all sides are crisp.

Toast the quinoa in a saucepan over medium-low flame for 5 minutes while constantly stirring. Turn the heat to low and add the broth. Cover the pan and simmer for 15 minutes. Fluff the cooked quinoa using a fork.

Mix the sauce in a heatproof bowl. Put the peanut butter and microwave for 10 seconds or until melted. Stir in the remaining ingredients and whisk to combine. Put the veggies, toasted almonds, herbs, tofu, and quinoa in a bowl. Add the sauce and mix well.

Crustless Quiche with Cheese

This recipe contains 19.5 grams of protein, 9 grams of fat, 3.6 grams of carbohydrates, and 176 calories per serving size of 1/8 of the recipe.

Here are the necessary ingredients to make 8 servings of the dish:

- 1 cup of skim milk

- 6 ounces of chicken breast, cut into cubes and grilled

- 3 eggs

- Non-stick cooking spray

- 4 ounces of low-fat Baby Swiss, cut into cubes

- Oregano as seasoning

- 10 ounces of shredded low-fat mozzarella cheese

Lay the baby Swiss and chicken breast in a pie pan. Add the shredded mozzarella cheese on top and sprinkle with oregano. Whisk the eggs and skim milk in a bowl. Pour this on top of the pan. Bake for 40 minutes in a preheated oven at 400 degrees. Leave to cool before serving.

12 - Bariatric-Friendly Seafood and Vegetables Recipes

Healthy Tuna Patty

This recipe contains 12 grams of protein, 1 gram of fat, 4 grams of carbohydrates, and 80 calories per serving size of 1/8 of the recipe.

To make 8 servings of the dish, you will need the following ingredients:

- 1 tablespoon of chopped onion

- 4 egg whites

- 16 crushed crackers

- 1/4 cup each of diced red pepper, capers, and chopped water chestnuts

- 4 3-ounce cans of tuna in water

- Dill, pepper, and dried mustard to taste

The first step is to put all the ingredients in a bowl. Mix well. Divide them into 8 and shape each into a patty. Cook the patties in a greased skillet over medium heat until both sides are browned.

You can opt to serve this along with 1 spoon of fat-free Greek yogurt.

Broiled Orange Roughy

This recipe contains 17 grams of protein, 4 grams of fat, 3 grams of carbohydrates, and 114 calories per serving size of 1 cup.

Here are the ingredients that you will need to make 4 servings of this dish:

- 1 tablespoon each of Dijon mustard and olive oil

- 8 lemon wedges

- 3 tablespoons of lemon juice

- 1/4 teaspoon of ground pepper

- 16 ounces of orange roughy fillets

Combine the lemon juice, ground pepper, olive oil, and

mustard in a bowl. Pu the fillets on a baking sheet that is lined with greased foil. Brush the fish with half of the lemon juice. Broil for 5 minutes. Drizzle the rest of the lemon juice on top of the broiled fillets. Top with the lemon wedges and season with pepper before serving.

Cheesy Broccoli with Egg

This recipe contains 12 grams of protein, 5 grams of fat, 5 grams of carbohydrates, and 115 calories per serving size of 1 slice.

The following ingredients are needed to make 8 servings of the dish:

- 6 eggs

- 1/2 cup of sliced mushrooms

- 10 ounces of chopped broccoli

- 1 teaspoon of salt

- 1/2 pound of low-fat cheddar cheese

- 6 tablespoons of flour

- 2 pounds of nonfat cottage cheese

- 1 4-ounce jar of chopped pimento

- A dash each of black pepper and paprika

This is easy to do. Simply mix all the ingredients in a bowl. Transfer the mixture to a greased pan. Bake for 90 minutes in a preheated oven at 350 degrees.

This is best eaten while hot.

Vegetarian Pizza with Ranch Dressing

This recipe contains 10 grams of protein, 10 grams of fat, 12 grams of carbohydrates, and 170 calories per serving size of 1/4 tortilla.

Prepare the following ingredients to make 4 servings of this healthy snack:

- 1/8 cup of shredded carrots

- 1 pack of dry mix ranch dressing

- 1/2 cup of low-fat chive and onion cream cheese

- 1/2 cup of light sour cream

- 3/4 cup each of shredded Colby & Monterey Jack cheese, diced tomatoes, and raw broccoli

- 2 large low-carb tortilla wraps

- 1/8 cup each of diced green pepper and diced cucumber

Put the packet of ranch dressing in a bowl. Mix it with cream cheese and sour cream. Lay the tortillas and spread them with the mixture. Add the vegetables and olives on top, plus a generous heap of cheese. Slice each to tortilla into 4 before serving.

Pureed Cauliflower

This recipe contains 5 grams of protein, 6 grams of fat, 13 grams of carbohydrates, and 113 calories per serving size of 3/4 cup.

To make 4 serving of the dish, you will need the following:

- 1/3 cup of low-fat buttermilk

- 1 teaspoon of salted butter

- 3 garlic cloves

- 4 teaspoons of extra-virgin olive oil

- 1/2 teaspoon each of garlic salt and black pepper

- 1 large cauliflower head

First, steam the cauliflower head along with the garlic cloves. Chop the cauliflower into small pieces and put them in a heatproof bowl. Add the garlic cloves and 1/4 cup of water. Cover the bowl before putting it inside the microwave oven. Steam in the microwave for 5 minutes on a high setting.

Put the steamed garlic cloves in the food processor and process until crushed. Add the buttermilk, steamed cauliflower, pepper, 2 teaspoons of olive oil, butter, and garlic salt. Process until the mixture looks creamy.

Transfer to a serving bowl and drizzle with the remaining olive oil before serving.

French Toast with Stuffing

This recipe contains 25 grams of protein, 0.5 gram of fat, 27 grams of carbohydrates, and 227 calories per serving.

The following ingredients will yield a serving of this recipe:

- 4 slices of low-calorie bread

- 3 egg whites

- 1/4 teaspoon of pumpkin pie spice

- 2 packets of sugar substitute

- A dash each of salt and vanilla

- 1/2 cup of fat-free ricotta cheese

Lay 2 slices of bread and spread them with ricotta cheese. Sprinkle them with the sugar substitute. Cover each slice with the remaining bread slices.

Whisk the egg whites on a bowl. Add salt, vanilla, and 1/4 teaspoon of pumpkin pie spice. Mix well. Dip the sandwiches into the mixture. Fry them in a greased skillet over medium heat until both sides are browned.

Vegetarian Chili with Cheese

This recipe contains 13 grams of protein, 3 grams of fat, 34 grams of carbohydrates, and 195 calories per serving size of 1 1/2 cups.

To make 8 servings of this dish, you will need the following:

- 8 ounces of tomato sauce

- 1 14.5-ounce can of diced tomatoes

- 1 zucchini (sliced)

- 2 garlic cloves

- 1/2 pound of mushrooms (sliced)

- 2 tablespoons of chili powder

- 1 10-ounce pack of frozen corn

- 2 15-ounce cans of red kidney beans (rinsed and drained)

- 1 green bell pepper (chopped)

- 1 cup of chopped onion

- 2 teaspoons of olive oil

- 1 cup of shredded low-fat cheddar cheese

Heat pan over medium-high flame. Add oil. Put the garlic once the oil is heated and sauté for a couple of minutes. Stir in the onions, pepper, and mushrooms, and cook for 3 minutes. Add the tomato sauce, diced tomatoes, and chili powder. Simmer for 15 minutes. Stir in the fresh corn and half a cup of the cheese. Simmer for 15 more minutes. Sprinkle cheddar cheese on top before serving.

Broccoli Quiche with Tofu

This recipe contains 13 grams of protein, 8 grams of fat, 18 grams of carbohydrates, and 190 calories per serving size of 1/6 of the recipe.

Here are the ingredients that you will need to make 6 servings of the dish:

- 1 yellow onion (sliced)

- 1 1/2 pounds of tofu

- A pinch of salt

- 2 tablespoons of sesame tahini

- 1/2 cup of uncooked bulgur wheat

- 1/2 pound of broccoli (chopped)

- 1 tablespoon each of sesame oil, white miso, and tamari

- 1/4 pound of mushrooms (chopped)

Put 1 cup of water in a pot over medium-high heat. Once it boils, add salt and the bulgur. Bring to another boil. Lower the heat and cover the pot. Simmer for 15 minutes. Put the cooked bulgur into an oiled pie pan. Press to make it firm. Bake for 12 minutes in a preheated oven at 350 degrees. Set this aside.

Heat oil in a skillet over medium-high flame. Put the onions, broccoli, and mushrooms. Sauté for 2 minutes.

Cover the skillet and remove from heat. Set this aside.

Put the tamari, white miso, tofu, and tahini in a food processor. Process until smooth.

Transfer the cooked vegetables in a bowl. Add the tofu mixture and toss to combine. Transfer them to the bulgur crust. Bake for 30 minutes. Allow to cool for 10 minutes before slicing into 6 pieces.

Ratatouille

This recipe contains 4.5 grams of protein, 2 grams of fat, 9 grams of carbohydrates, and 335 calories per serving.

The following ingredients will yield 4 servings of this healthy recipe:

- 1 red capsicum (diced)

- 2 zucchinis (diced)

- 1 onion (chopped)

- 1 garlic clove (crushed)

- 1 eggplant (diced)

- 1 stick of celery (diced)

- 400 grams of tomatoes (chopped and with no added salt)

- Oil spray

- 1/4 cup of fresh basil (chopped)

- 2 cups of mushrooms (diced)

Lightly grease a pan over medium heat. Cook the onion and garlic for a couple of minutes. Add the celery, mushrooms, and capsicum, and sauté for 4 minutes. Transfer to a plate and set aside.

Spray the same pan with a bit of oil. Cook the zucchinis and eggplant until soft. Stir in the basil and basil, and put back the mushroom mixture. Lower the heat and simmer for 5 minutes.

Freeze any leftover and reheat when needed.

Shrimp Ceviche

This recipe contains 25 grams of protein, 1 gram of fat, 13 grams of carbohydrates, and 160 calories per serving size of 4 ounces.

Here are the needed ingredients to make 4 servings of this dish:

- 2 serrano chili peppers (minced)

- 3/4 cup of red onion (chopped)

- 1 pound of raw shrimp

- 1 cup of lime juice

- 1 bunch of cilantro (chopped)

- 4 tomatoes (diced)

Put the shrimp in a bowl. Drizzle with lime juice. Make sure that all the pieces of shrimp are covered with the juice. Cover the bowl and leave for 15 minutes to marinate.

Take note of the time. Do not marinate the shrimp for more

than 15 minutes because they will become tough. Add the onions, tomatoes, cilantro, and chili peppers, and mix well until combined. Season with salt and pepper before serving.

Black Bean with Pumpkin Soup

This recipe contains 15 grams of protein, 6 grams of fat, 46 grams of carbohydrates, and 290 calories per serving size of 1 cup.

You will need the following ingredients to make 6 servings of this dish:

- 1 16-ounce can of pumpkin puree

- 2 15-ounce cans of black beans (rinsed and drained)

- 1 cup of diced tomatoes (canned)

- 2 cups of beef broth

- 4 garlic cloves (chopped)

- 1/2 teaspoon of black pepper

- 2 tablespoons of olive oil

- 1 tablespoon of ground cumin

- 1 teaspoon of chili powder

- 1 onion (chopped)

Put oil in a pan over medium heat. Cook the onion and garlic for a couple of minutes. Season with the cumin, chili powder, and pepper. Stir in the tomatoes, black beans, and pumpkin. Add the broth. Simmer for 25 minutes while occasionally stirring. You can serve the soup as is or puree using an immersion blender.

Black Bean and Corn Salad

This recipe contains 6 grams of protein, 5 grams of fat, 23 grams of carbohydrates, and 160 calories per serving size of 1/2 cup.

Prepare the following ingredients to make 6 servings of this dish:

- 1/4 teaspoon of ground black pepper

- 2 16-ounce cans of black beans, rinsed and drained

- 2 tablespoons each of olive oil and minced red onion

- 1 cup of whole kernel corn

- A dash of salt

- 1 teaspoon each of minced garlic, lemon juice and brown sugar

- 1/4 cup each of balsamic vinegar and chopped fresh parsley

Put the fresh corn, black beans, red onion, and fresh parsley in a bowl and mix. In another bowl, mix the honey, garlic, balsamic vinegar, olive oil, salt and pepper, and lemon juice. Mix until combined. Combine the 2 mixtures. Leave for 30 minutes before serving.

Spicy Peanut Vegetarian Chili

This recipe contains 8 grams of protein, 2.5 grams of fat, 22 grams of carbohydrates, and 125 calories per serving size of 1/2 cup.

Here are the needed ingredients to make 12 servings of this

dish:

- 2 tablespoons of chili powder

- 1 28-ounce can of diced tomato

- 1 16-ounce can each of white beans and white beans, rinsed and drained

- 1 cup of chopped onion

- 1 15-ounce can of tomato sauce

- 2 garlic cloves, minced

- 2 cups of vegetable broth

- 1/4 teaspoon of dried oregano

- 1 tablespoon of peanut oil

- 1 teaspoon of chipotle chili pepper

- 1/3 cup of powdered peanuts

Heat oil in a pot over medium-high flame. Add the onion and garlic. Cook for 4 minutes. Stir in the chili powder, salt, pepper, and oregano. Sauté for 2 minutes. Add the beans, tomato sauce, corn, tomatoes, powdered peanuts, and broth. Stir the ingredients. Bring it to a boil. Turn the heat to low and leave for 30 minutes to simmer.

13 - Bariatric-Friendly Meat Recipes

Chicken with Peanut and Applesauce

This recipe contains 3 grams of protein, 2 grams of fat, 13 grams of carbohydrates, and 50 calories per serving size of 2 tablespoons.

The following ingredients will yield 8 servings of this dish:

- 2 1/2 pounds of sliced chicken

- 1/4 cup of yellow mustard

- 1 15-ounce jar of unsweetened applesauce

- Salt and pepper to taste

- 1/8 cup of unpacked Splenda brown sugar

- 1/2 cup of powdered peanuts

Heat pan over medium-high flame. Put the meat and saute for a couple of minutes. Add the brown sugar, peanuts, mustard, and applesauce. Stir the ingredients until combined. Reduce the heat to medium. Simmer for 10 minutes.

Chicken Cheesesteak Wrap

This recipe contains 33 grams of protein, 6 grams of fat, 17 grams of carbohydrates, and 264 calories per serving size of 1 wrap.

You will need the following ingredients to make a serving of this dish:

- 1 whole wheat low-carb tortilla

- 1/4 pound of skinless and boneless chicken breast, with the visible fat trimmed and thinly sliced into strips

- 1 3/4-ounce wedge of light Swiss cheese

- 1/4 cup each of chopped onions, sliced green pepper, and sliced mushrooms

- 2 teaspoons of sliced pickled hot chili peppers

Heat oil in a skillet over medium flame. Cook the onion and meat until done. Stir in the green peppers and mushroom. Cook for 4 minutes. Lay the tortilla in the middle of 2 moist paper towels. Microwave for 20 seconds on a high setting.

Add a strip of cheese in the middle. Put the chicken, onions, peppers, mushrooms, and onions on top. Add chili peppers if you want it to be spicier. Fold the tortilla before serving.

Chicken Taco Filling

This recipe contains 23 grams of protein, 2.4 grams of fat, 6 grams of carbohydrates, and 148 calories per serving size of 4 ounces.

To make 4 servings of this dish, you will need the following:

- 1 pound of skinless and boneless chicken breasts

- 1 cup of chicken broth

- 1 1.25-ounce pack of dry taco seasoning mix

Put the chicken broth in a bowl and mix it with the taco seasoning. Place the meat in a slow cooker. Pour the seasoning mixture over the meat. Lock the lid in place and cook for 8 hours. Shred the chicken and continue cooking for 30 minutes.

Use the cooked mixture as filling for tacos or as toppings for salads.

Baked Chicken and Veggies

This recipe contains 26 grams of protein, 3.5 grams of fat, 25 grams of carbohydrates, and 240 calories per serving size of 1/6 of the recipe.

Here are the necessary ingredients to make 6 servings of the dish:

- 1 raw chicken, skinless and cut into bite-size pieces

- 6 carrots, sliced

- 1 teaspoon of thyme

- 4 potatoes, sliced

- 1/2 cup of water

- 1 onion, quartered

- 1/4 teaspoon of pepper

Lay the potatoes, onions, and carrots at the bottom of a large roasting pan. Place the meat on top. In a bowl, mix water, pepper, and thyme. Add the mixture to the pan. Bake in a preheated oven at 400 degrees for 1 hour. Twice during the process, get the pan from the oven and spoon over the juices on top. Bake until the meat is tender.

Chicken Caprese

This recipe contains 33 grams of protein, 9 grams of fat, 4 grams of carbohydrates, and 230 calories per serving size of 1 ounce each of cheese and tomato, and 4 ounces of chicken.

Prepare the following ingredients to make 4 servings of this dish:

- 3 tablespoons of balsamic vinegar

- 1 pound of skinless and boneless chicken breasts

- 1 tablespoon of olive oil

- 1 ripe tomato, quartered

- Pepper, to taste

- 2 tablespoons of thinly sliced basil

- 4 slices of fresh mozzarella cheese

- 1 teaspoon of dry Italian seasoning

Put the meat in a bowl and season with oil, pepper, and dry Italian seasoning. Put the seasoned meat on a preheated grill over medium-high heat. Grill each side for 5 minutes or until well-done. Sprinkle the mozzarella cheese on top. Cook for 1 more minute before transferring to a plate. Top each piece of meat with pepper, basil, 1 slice of tomato and balsamic vinegar before serving.

Creamy Chicken in Slow Cooker

This recipe contains 18.5 grams of protein, 1.68 grams of fat, and 128 calories per serving size of 6 ounces.

Here are the necessary ingredients to make 6 servings of the dish:

- 1/2 cup of chicken stock

- 1 cup of plain Greek yogurt

- 1 8-ounce pack of mushrooms

- 2.5 pounds of skinless and boneless chicken breasts

- 1 7-ounce envelope of Italian dressing mix

- 1 10-ounce can of low-fat cream of mushroom soup

Heat a greased skillet over medium-high flame. Cook the meat in batches until browned. Put the browned meat in a slow cooker. Pour the soup into the same skillet. Add the Italian dressing mix, chicken stock, and yogurt.

Stir the mixture until combined. Pour the soup over the meat in the slow cooker. Add the mushrooms. Lock the lid in place and cook for 4 hours on low setting. Stir the soup before serving.

Brown Rice and Beans Casserole

This recipe contains 31 grams of protein, 6 grams of fat, 22 grams of carbohydrates, and 267 calories per serving size of 1/8 of the recipe.

Prepare the following ingredients to make 8 servings of this dish:

- 1 4-ounce can of green chilies, diced

- 16 ounces of skinless and boneless chicken breasts,

chopped

- 1/2 teaspoon of cumin

- 1 cup of vegetable broth

- 1 tablespoon of olive oil

- 1/3 cup each of brown rice and diced onion

- 1 zucchini, sliced

- 1 15-ounce can of black beans, drained

- 1/3 cup of shredded carrots

- 2 cups shredded low-fat Swiss cheese

- 1/4 teaspoon of cayenne pepper

- 1/2 cup of sliced mushrooms

Mix the rice and broth in a pot over medium-high flame. Bring to a boil. Cover the pot and reduce the heat to low. Simmer for 45 minutes or until the rice is tender. Heat oil in a skillet over medium flame. Put the onion and sauté for 3 minutes. Stir in the zucchini, seasonings, mushrooms, and meat. Cook for 5 minutes.

Transfer the cooked rice to a bowl. Pour over the cooked meat and zucchini mixture. Add the chilies, carrots, beans, and 1 cup of Swiss cheese. Mix thoroughly until combined. Transfer the mixture to an oiled casserole dish.

Sprinkle the remaining cheese on top. Cover the casserole dish with loose foil. Bake for half an hour in a preheated oven at 350 degrees. Remove the foil and continue baking for 10 more minutes.

Chicken with Greek Yogurt

This recipe contains 46 grams of protein, 4 grams of fat, 3 grams of carbohydrates, and 266 calories per serving size of 1 cup.

Here are the needed ingredients to make 4 servings of this dish:

- 4 skinless and boneless chicken breasts

- 1 cup of plain Greek yogurt

- 1/2 cup of grated Parmesan cheese

- 1 1/2 teaspoons of salt

- 1 teaspoon of garlic powder

- 1/2 teaspoon of pepper

Mix the Greek yogurt, seasonings, and cheese in a bowl. Season the meat with the mixture. Arrange the coated meat on a greased baking sheet lined with foil. Bake for 45 minutes in a preheated oven at 375 degrees.

Southwest Pasta Salad with Chicken

This recipe contains 21 grams of protein, 9.9 grams of fat, 38.2 grams of carbohydrates, and 322 calories per serving size of 1 1/3 cups.

The following ingredients will yield 6 servings of this dish:

- 1/2 pound of uncooked penne rigate

- 1 cup of fresh corn kernels

- 2 cups of skinless and boneless lemon-herb chicken, grilled

- 1 tablespoon each of extra-virgin olive oil and canned

chipotle chili in adobo, chopped

- 1/2 teaspoon of salt

- 2 tablespoons of fresh lime juice

- 1/2 cup each of diced red bell pepper, chopped plum tomato, and sliced green onions

- 1/4 cup of fresh orange juice

- 3 ounces of shredded sharp cheddar cheese

Remove the fat and salt from the package of the penne rigate and cook according to instructions. Drain the liquid. Put the cooked pasta in a bowl. Add the corn kernels, red bell pepper, meat, cheese, green onions, and tomato.

Toss the ingredients until combined. Mix all the remaining ingredients in another bowl. Pour this over the pasta mixture and gently toss. Cover the bowl and leave in the fridge for at least 30 minutes before serving.

Faux Fried Chicken

This recipe contains 29 grams of protein, 3.5 grams of fat,

17 grams of carbohydrates, and 210 calories per serving size of 3 pieces.

You will need the following ingredients to make 3 servings of this dish:

- 1/3 cup each of panko breadcrumbs, bran cereal, and reduced-fat buttermilk

- 12 ounces of skinless and boneless lean chicken breasts

- Salt to taste

- 1 tablespoon of dry onion soup mix

- 1/8 teaspoon of paprika

Mix the buttermilk and paprika in a bag. Put the meat. Seal the bag and shake until all sides of the meat is coated with the mixture. Refrigerate for 1 hour. Process the cereal in the food processor until it has the same consistency as breadcrumbs. Transfer to a bowl.

Add the panko breadcrumbs and onion soup. Mix until combined. Season with salt. Coat the meat with the mixture and arrange all pieces on an oiled baking sheet. Bake for 10 minutes in a preheated oven at 375 degrees. Flip the meat and continue baking for 10 more minutes.

Super Moist Chicken

This recipe contains 37 grams of protein, 5 grams of fat, 8 grams of carbohydrates, and 233 calories per serving size of 1 cup.

To make 12 servings of this dish, you will need the following:

- 1 1/4 cups of whole wheat Italian bread crumbs

- 1/2 cup of light mayo of choice

- 3 pounds of skinless and boneless chicken breasts

Brush all sides of the meat with light mayo. Roll the coated meat in bread crumbs and arrange them in a pan lined with foil. Bake for 45 minutes in a preheated oven at 425 degrees.

Chicken Casserole

This recipe contains 19 grams of protein, 8 grams of fat, 27 grams of carbohydrates, and 256 calories per serving size of 1 cup.

Here are the necessary ingredients to make 4 servings of the dish:

- 2 cups of frozen mixed vegetables

- 1 cup of skinless and boneless chicken breast, cooked

- 1 cup of 2 percent milk

- 4 ounces of canned mushrooms

- 1 cup of shredded cheddar cheese

- 1/2 cup of uncooked whole wheat pasta

- 3/4 cup of water

- Pepper, onion powder, and garlic powder to taste

- 1 10.5-ounce can of fat-free cream of chicken soup

Cook the pasta and veggies according to package directions. Transfer them to a bowl. Add the chicken, mushrooms, water, soup, 1/2 cup of cheese, and milk. Season with garlic powder, pepper, and onion powder. Stir until mixed. Transfer to a greased casserole dish. Add the rest of the cheese on top. Bake for 30 minutes in a preheated oven at 350 degrees.

Chicken Tetrazzini

This recipe contains 10 grams of protein, 3 grams of fat, 25 grams of carbohydrates, and 167 calories per serving size of 1 cup.

Prepare the following ingredients to make 6 servings of this dish:

- 1 cup of fat-free chicken broth

- 1/2 pound of skinless and boneless chicken breasts, cooked and cut into cubes

- 1/2 cup of chopped scallions

- 3 tablespoons of all-purpose flour

- 8 ounces of sliced button mushrooms

- 8 ounces of spaghetti, split into thirds and cooked

- 1/2 cup of fat-free skim milk

- 1 tablespoon of low-calorie margarine

- 2 tablespoons of sherry cooking wine

- 1/4 cup of pimentos, drained and chopped

- 1/4 teaspoon of garlic powder

- 1/8 teaspoon of black pepper

- 3 1/2 tablespoons of grated Parmesan cheese

Melt the margarine in a pan over medium-high heat. Add the scallions and mushrooms. Saute for 5 minutes while stirring frequently. In a bowl, combine the flour, garlic powder, broth, milk, and pepper.

Add this to the pan and cook until it boils. Keep on stirring the mixture until thick. Add the chicken, pimientos, and sherry. Cook for 2 more minutes while occasionally stirring. Add the cheese and cooked spaghetti. Toss the ingredients until combined.

Black Bean Verde and Pork Stew

This recipe contains 33 grams of protein, 7 grams of fat, 25 grams of carbohydrates, and 308 calories per serving size of 1/4 of the recipe.

Here are the needed ingredients to make 4 servings of this dish:

- 3 garlic cloves

- 1 teaspoon each of ground cumin and crushed red pepper flakes

- 1 pound of pork tenderloin, trim the visible fat and cut into cubes

- 2 teaspoons of extra-virgin olive oil

- 1 seasoning packet

- 2 chipotle peppers canned in adobo sauce, minced, plus 1 teaspoon of the sauce

- 1 1/4 cups of chopped onions

- 1 14.5-ounce of diced tomatoes with no salt added

- 1 14.5-ounce of black beans with no added salt, rinsed and drained

- 1 14-ounce can of chicken broth with no salt added

Put olive oil in a pot over medium-high heat. Once the oil is heated, add the meat and cook until all sides are browned. Stir in the onion and garlic. Cook for 3 more minutes. Add the cumin, chipotle sauce, sauce, and seasoning packet. Mix well. Stir in the tomatoes, beans, red pepper flakes, and broth. Bring to a boil. Reduce the heat to low and cover the pot. Continue cooking for 1 hour.

You can eat the soup as is or pour it over brown rice. Adjust the nutritional content of the dish if you will opt for the latter.

Sweet and Sour Pork Recipe

This recipe contains 18 grams of protein, 3.5 grams of fat, 348 grams of carbohydrates, and 248 calories per serving size of 1/2 cup of rice and 1 cup of the meat mixture.

The following ingredients will yield 6 servings of this dish:

- 3 cups of cooked brown rice

- 2 green peppers, chopped

- 1 15-ounce can of unsweetened pineapple chunks, drained and the juice reserved

- 1 pound of lean pork tenderloin, sliced into thin strips

- 1 onion, chopped

- 2 tablespoons of cornstarch

- 1/4 cup of Splenda brown sugar blend

- 1 tablespoon of low-sodium soy sauce

- 1/2 cup of water

- 1/3 cup of wine vinegar

- 1/2 teaspoon of salt

Heat a greased skillet over medium-high flame. Put the meat and cook until browned. Transfer to a plate and set aside. In a bowl, mix the vinegar, sugar, soy sauce, salt, water, reserved pineapple juice, and cornstarch. Remove the oil from the same skillet and add the mixture.

Cook for 2 minutes while stirring constantly. Put the meat back to the skillet. Reduce the heat to low. Cook for half an hour while stirring every now and then. Stir in the peppers, onion, and pineapple chunks. Cook for 5 minutes. Pour the dish over cooked brown rice and serve.

Asian Pork Tenderloin

This recipe contains 10 grams of protein, 9 grams of fat, 9 grams of carbohydrates, and 256 calories per serving size of 4 ounces.

You will need the following ingredients to make 8 servings of this dish:

- 4 garlic cloves, minced

- 1 1/2 teaspoons of pepper

- 2 pounds of pork tenderloin

- 2 tablespoons each of Worcestershire sauce, lemon juice, dry mustard, and rice vinegar

- 1/3 cup each of brown sugar and light soy sauce

- 1 tablespoon each of ginger and dry mustard

Combine all the ingredients, except the meat, in a freezer bag. Shake well before adding the meat. Seal the bag. Put in the fridge overnight to marinate. The next day, cook the marinated meat in a slow cooker for 6 hours. You can also opt to bake it instead for 40 minutes in a preheated oven at 375 degrees.

Whopper Veggie Burger

This recipe contains 18 grams of protein, 5.5 grams of fat, 40 grams of carbohydrates, and 260 calories per serving size.

To make a serving of this dish, you will need the following:

Onion, Lettuce, and Tomato

- 1 whole wheat hamburger bun

- 1 tablespoon each of ketchup, mustard, and light mir-acle whip

- 1 savory mushroom mozzarella-flavored Boca Burger

Cook the Boca Burger according to package directions. Use this as filling of a bun. Lay the other ingredients on top, such as the onion, lettuce, ketchup, tomato, and light miracle whip. If you have more time in your hands, you can whip up your own burger by using lean ground turkey breast or ground beef.

Ginger Beef Stir Fry Recipe

This recipe contains 17 grams of protein, 8 grams of fat, 25 grams of carbohydrates, and 275 calories per serving size of 1/6 of the recipe.

Here are the necessary ingredients to make 6 servings of the dish:

- 6 ounces of fat-free beef broth

- 1 pound of flank steak, sliced

- 2 garlic cloves

- 1 teaspoon of canola oil

- 1 8-ounce can of water chestnuts, sliced

- 1 tablespoon of cornstarch

- 1/4 teaspoon of crushed red pepper flakes

- 2 teaspoons of ground ginger

- 1/2 cup of instant brown rice

- 3 tablespoons of soy sauce

- 2 ounces of hoisin sauce

- 1/2 bell pepper, sliced

- 3 ounces of broccoli florets

- 2 stalks of bok choy, sliced

Put the meat in a bowl. Season it with ginger and garlic. Cook the rice according to directions. In a bowl, combine the cornstarch, hoisin sauce, broth, and soy sauce. Heat a skillet over medium-high flame. Add oil. Cook the meat and red pepper flakes for 5 minutes while constantly stirring.

In another pan over medium-high flame, put the broccoli,

carrot, and bell pepper. Sauté for 3 minutes while stirring frequently. You can add up to 2 tablespoons of water if you find the mixture too dry.

Add the bok choy and water chestnuts. Cook for 2 minutes while stirring often. Add the broth and cook for 2 more minutes while stirring constantly. Add the beef and cook for 2 more minutes. Pour this over the rice and serve.

Turkey Turnover Recipe

This recipe contains 9 grams of protein, 7 grams of fat, 13 grams of carbohydrates, and 155 calories per serving size of 2 pieces.

Prepare the following ingredients to make 24 servings of this dish:

- 1 envelope of dry onion soup

- 1 pound of ground turkey breast meat

- 3 tubes of low-fat refrigerated crescent rolls

- 1 cup of shredded low-fat cheese

Heat soup in a skillet over medium-high flame. Add the meat. Cook until the meat is browned while occasionally stirring. Stir in the cheese and mix until combined. Turn the heat off and set aside.

Separate the rolls and slice each piece of the triangle in half. Scoop 1 tablespoon of the meat mixture to each half of the roll. Fold the dough and seal. Arrange them on a greased cookie sheet. Bake for 15 minutes in a preheated oven at 350 degrees.

Turkey Bean Enchilada Recipe

This recipe contains 14 grams of protein, 3 grams of fat, 19 grams of carbohydrates, and 175 calories per serving size of 1 enchilada.

Here are the needed ingredients to make 4 servings of this dish:

- 4 fat-free tortillas

- 2 cups of skinless white turkey meat, cooked and cut into cubes

- 1 15-ounce can of pinto beans, rinsed and drained

- 1/2 cup of shredded low-fat Mexican cheese

- 1 cup of canned enchilada sauce, divided

- 6 scallions, green and white parts only, chopped

Put the scallions, turkey, beans, and 1/2 cup of enchilada sauce in a bowl. Mix until combined. Scoop 1/4 of the mixture to each tortilla. Fold the top, bottom, and sides of the tortilla to envelope the filling. Put them in a baking dish. Pour the remaining sauce on top and add cheese. Cover the pan. Bake for 20 minutes in a preheated oven at 350 degrees.

Zucchini Boat

This recipe contains 17.5 grams of protein, 7.5 grams of fat, 16 grams of carbohydrates, and 195 calories per serving size of 1 piece.

The following ingredients will yield 8 servings of this dish:

- 1 beaten egg

- 4 zucchinis, sliced in half lengthwise

- 1 pound of ground turkey breast

- 1/2 cup of chopped onion

- 3/4 cup of spaghetti sauce

- 1/4 teaspoon each of pepper and salt

- 1/4 cup of seasoned whole wheat bread crumbs

- 1 tomato, chopped

- 1/2 pound of sliced mushrooms

- 4 ounces of low-fat Mozzarella cheese

Thinly cut the bottom of each zucchini slice and scoop out the pulp. Set the pulp aside. Arrange the shells in a heat-proof dish. Cover the dish for 3 minutes on a high setting. Remove the liquid and set aside. Cook the meat and onion in a skillet over medium flame.

Once the meat is well-done, remove from heat and drain the liquid. Put this in a bowl and add the breadcrumbs, beaten egg, spaghetti sauce, 1/2 cup of cheese, zucchini pulp, mushrooms, and tomato. Mix until combined. Scoop 1/4 of the mixture into each zucchini shell. Bake for 20 minutes in a preheated oven at 350 degrees.

Stuffed Cabbage Rolls Recipe

This recipe contains 15 grams of protein, 5.5 grams of fat, 16 grams of carbohydrates, and 174 calories per serving size of 1 roll.

You will need the following ingredients to make 6 servings of this dish:

- 1/3 cup of preferred whole grain rice

- 1 pound of 93 percent lean ground turkey

- 1 cabbage head, separate the leaves, wash, and blanch for 30 seconds

- 1 teaspoon of olive oil

- 2 teaspoons each of Italian seasoning and garlic powder

- 2 carrots, diced

- 1/2 onion, diced

- 2 cups of tomato sauce

Cook the rice according to package directions. Heat a skillet over medium flame. Add the olive oil. Saute the onions and carrots for 3 minutes while stirring often. Add the meat and cook until browned. Add the powders and seasonings. Mix well. Pour this over the cooked rice.

Mix thoroughly until combined. Scoop 1/2 of the mixture in every cabbage leaf. Roll the leaf to wrap the filling and seal the ends. Put them in a baking dish. Pour over the tomato sauce. Bake for 45 minutes in a preheated oven at 350 degrees. Set aside to cool for 5 minutes before serving.

14 - Bariatric-Friendly Recipes for Sauces, Spreads and Desserts

Squash Apple Bake

This recipe contains 1 gram of protein, 8 grams of fat, 17 grams of carbohydrates, and 133 calories per serving size of 1/6 of the recipe.

To make 6 servings of this dish, you will need the following:

- 2 teaspoons of ground cinnamon

- 2 apples, peeled, cored and sliced

- 1 tablespoon each of all-purpose flour and Splenda

- 1/2 teaspoon of salt

- 1/4 cup of melted butter

- 1 butternut squash, peeled and cubed

Mix the squash and apples in a casserole dish. Put the remaining ingredients in a bowl and mix well. Add this to the casserole dish and mix all the ingredients until combined. Cover the casserole dish. Bake for 50 minutes in a preheated oven at 350 degrees. Remove the cover and continue baking for 10 more minutes.

Creamy Jell-O

This recipe contains 1 gram of protein, 2 grams of carbohydrates, and 30 calories per serving size of 1/2 cup.

You will need the following ingredients to make 4 servings of this dish:

- 1 box of sugar-free Jell-O

- 8 tablespoons of Cool Whip Free

Prepare the Jell-O according to package instructions. Put in the fridge until set. Divide the set gelatin into 4 cups. Add 2 tablespoons of Cool Whip Free into each cup. Stir the ingredients in every cup and serve.

Chocolate Soy

This recipe contains 5 grams of protein, 1 gram of fat, 6 grams of carbohydrates, and 56 calories per serving size of 1/2 cup.

14 - BARIATRIC-FRIENDLY RECIPES FOR SAUCES, SPREADS AND DESSERTS

The following ingredients will yield 8 servings of this dish:

- 1/4 cup of hot water

- 1 packet of unflavored gelatin

- 1 1.4-ounce pack of fat-free and sugar-free chocolate fudge instant pudding

- 1 cup of cold skim milk

- 16 ounces of silken tofu, cut into cubes

- 1 tablespoon of cocoa powder

- 1/4 teaspoon of peppermint extract

- 1/2 teaspoon of vanilla extract

Dissolve the gelatin in hot water. Stir thoroughly so that no lumps are formed. Put in the fridge until set. In a bowl, combine the skim milk and instant pudding mix. Add the diced tofu.

Break up the pieces of tofu as you whisk the mixture. Transfer to a food processor and process until smooth. Slowly add the gelatin and process until the consistency is the same as a smoothie. Transfer to a glass dish, cover and put in the fridge. Serve once firm.

Fluffy Cottage Cheese

This recipe contains 22 grams of protein, 3 grams of fat, 24 grams of carbohydrates, and 220 calories per serving size of 1 cup.

Here are the needed ingredients to make 8 servings of this dish:

- 2 24-ounce packs of fat-free cottage cheese

- 1 8-ounce pack of sugar-free whipped topping

- 2 0.3-ounce pack of sugar-free gelatin

Mix all the ingredients in a bowl and serve. You can also add any fruit to the mixture to tweak the taste and increase its nutrient content.

Spicy Avocado Spread

This recipe contains 2 grams of protein, 5 grams of fat, 8 grams of carbohydrates, and 85 calories per serving size of 4 tablespoons.

Prepare the following ingredients to make 6 servings of this dish:

- 1/2 teaspoon of green Tabasco sauce

- 2 sprigs of cilantro

- 1 1/2 tablespoons of fresh lime juice

- 1 ripe avocado

- 1/2 green jalapeño, with the seeds removed and chopped

- 2/3 cup of cannellini beans, drained and rinsed

- 1/4 teaspoon salt

Put all the ingredients in a food processor. Process until smooth and creamy. You can use this as dipping for vegetables or as chicken topping.

Yummy Pumpkin Mousse

This recipe contains 2 grams of protein, 4.4 grams of fat, 28 grams of carbohydrates, and 149 calories per serving size of 1 cup.

Here are the necessary ingredients to make 4 servings of the dish:

- 2 cups of sugar-free whipped topping

- 1 teaspoon of cinnamon

- 1 4-ounce pack of fat-free vanilla pudding

- Splenda, nutmeg, clove, allspice, and clove to taste

- 1/2 cup of skim milk

- 1 15-ounce can of pumpkin

Whisk all the ingredients in a bowl until creamy and smooth. Transfer to 4 cups and serve.

Peanut Powder Salad Dressing

This recipe contains 3 grams of protein, 2 grams of fat, 7 grams of carbohydrates, and 50 calories per serving size of 2 tablespoons.

To make 2 servings of this dish, you will need the following:

- 2 tablespoons of powdered peanuts

- 1 teaspoon of Splenda brown sugar blend

- 1/4 teaspoon each of Szechuan chili sauce and ground pepper

- 1/8 teaspoon each of sesame oil and garlic powder

- 1 tablespoon each of water and low-sodium soy sauce

Put all the ingredients in a food processor. Process until smooth.

Bean Spread

This recipe contains 11.5 grams of protein, 1.5 grams of fat, 34.5 grams of carbohydrates, and 198 calories per serving size of 2 tablespoons.

You will need the following ingredients to make 2 servings of this dish:

- 1 15-ounce can of pinto beans

- Salt and red or green Tabasco sauce, to taste

- Juice of 1 lime

Combine all the ingredients in a food processor and process until smooth.

Cucumber with Tzatziki Greek Yogurt Sauce

This recipe contains 6 grams of protein, 8 grams of carbohydrates, and 53 calories per serving size of 1 cup.

The following ingredients will yield 8-9 servings of this dish:

- 3 cups of fat-free plain Greek yogurt

- 2 cucumbers, peeled, seeded and chopped

- Salt and pepper to taste

- 3 tablespoons of lemon juice

- 1 garlic clove, minced

- 1 tablespoon each of salt and minced dill

Place the cucumber meat in a colander. Season with salt. Let stand for half an hour. Drain excess liquid and pat them with paper towels. Put all the seasoned cucumber pieces in a food processor. Add dill, garlic, lemon juice, and black pepper. Process until combined. Transfer to a bowl. Put in the fridge for at least 2 hours. Drain excess liquid before serving.

Balsamic Dijon Mustard Dressing

This recipe contains 0 gram of protein, 26 grams of carbohydrates, and 85 calories per serving size of 1 1/2 tablespoons.

Here are the needed ingredients to make 4 servings of this dish:

- 4 tablespoons of balsamic vinegar

- Pepper and oregano to taste

- 2 tablespoons Dijon mustard

Put all the ingredients in a bowl and mix well. You can use this as dressing for vegetables, chicken, or roasted salmon.

Protein Packed Pesto

This recipe contains 6 grams of protein, 5 grams of fat, 4 grams of carbohydrates, and 77 calories per serving size of 1/2 cup.

Prepare the following ingredients to make 4 servings of this dish:

- 2 garlic cloves, minced

- 1/2 cup of water

- 1/3 cup each of fresh basil and 1 percent cottage cheese

- 1 10-ounce pack of frozen spinach, thawed and

chopped

- 1 tablespoon of olive oil

- 2 tablespoons of grated Parmesan cheese

Combine all the ingredients in a food processor. Process until smooth. You can serve 1/2 cup of the sauce along with poultry or fish dishes.

Light Alfredo Sauce

This recipe contains 5 grams of protein, 4 grams of fat, 5 grams of carbohydrates, and 71 calories per serving size of 1/4 cup.

Here are the necessary ingredients to make 8 servings of the dish:

- 1/2 cup of grated Parmesan cheese

- 1/4 teaspoon of black pepper

- 2 cups of skim milk

- 1 tablespoon of extra virgin olive oil

- 1/2 teaspoon of salt

- 3 tablespoons of all-purpose flour

- 4 garlic cloves, minced

- 1 cup of warmed chicken broth

Put oil in a pan over medium flame. Put the garlic and cook for a couple of minutes. Add the flour and keep on stirring until thick. Add the chicken broth. Slowly whisk the mixture until combined.

Add milk and mix well. Season with salt and pepper. Reduce the heat to low. Keep on stirring until smooth and thick. Stir in the Parmesan cheese. You can use the sauce as topping for chicken, pasta, and fish dishes.

15 - Conclusion

Thank you again for buying this book!

I hope this book was able to help you understand the basics on how to help yourself recover from the gastric bypass surgery. Let this book be your guide to a fitter and healthier you.

The next step is to try out the recipes found in this book and plan your meals, especially after your Gastric Bypass Surgery.

Finally, if you enjoyed this book, then I'd like to ask you for a favor. Would you be kind enough to leave a review for this book on Amazon? It'd be greatly appreciated!

Book 2 - Bariatric Cookbook

Delicious Post Weight Loss Surgery Meal Plans (Coping Companion, Before & After, Lap Band, Keeping Skinny)

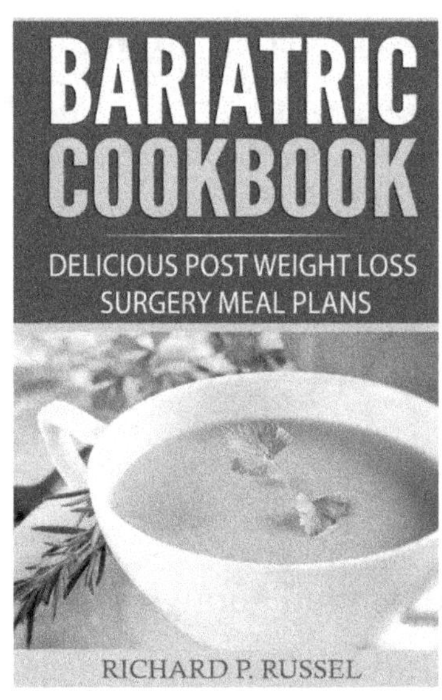

1 - Introduction

Over the years, morbid obesity has become a major issue in the United States and other developed countries. The numbers of people who are morbidly obese are rising. Morbidly obese people have a body mass index of 40 kg/m2 or more. Oftentimes, these people fail to lose weight using the conventional methods.

As a last resort, doctors recommend to these people gastric bypass surgery to help them combat obesity. The demand for gastric bypass surgery is increasing due to its effectiveness in helping morbidly obese people. Many obese people are successful in losing weight and in maintaining their ideal weight.

There are seven different types of gastric bypass surgeries. These are the adjustable gastric banding (or laparoscopic banding), gastric sleeve procedure, gastric pacing, gastric balloon, the classic Roux-en-Y or proximal gastric bypass, biliopancreatic diversion with duodenal switch and the Magenstrasse and Mill procedure

Each procedure entails a different way of bypassing the stomach. Generally, the goal is to alter the digestive system by reducing the capacity of the stomach. The "new stomach" can only hold 1/2 to 2 cups of food as compared to 6 cups of food that a normal stomach can digest.

The health condition of the person and urgency of performing the procedure will dictate the type of surgery that doctors will recommend.

Most of the surgeries are irreversible. You cannot undergo another surgery to bring back the old way your digestive system works. A gastric bypass surgery is a lifelong commitment. Commitment includes changing your lifestyle and eating habits.

2 - Understand Your Digestive System before the Surgery

The digestive system composes of nine essential body parts to complete the process. Digestion starts in the mouth. Your mouth breaks down food by chewing and releasing enzymes. The swallowed food passes through the esophagus and reaches the stomach. The stomach releases gastric acid to further break down the food.

Do you know that the stomach can hold a maximum of 6 cups in every meal? Yes, that is the size of a football. When the digestive system malfunctions, you can eat more than this capacity of your stomach.

The stomach signals the gallbladder and pancreas when it cannot break down certain types of components in the food. The gallbladder for an instance produces bile to help the stomach break down fat. The pancreas secretes insulin and other digestive enzymes to break down sugar in your food.

If the pancreas does not produce the right amount of insulin and digestive enzymes, the sugar in food is stored as fat. The pancreas can increase blood sugar levels, which may lead to diabetes if constant delays in breaking down the sugar reoccur too many times.

When the stomach finishes the churning of food, it transfers the food to the small intestines. The small intestines have three major parts, the duodenum, jejunum, and ileum. The food passes through the duodenum where many of the minerals and vitamins in the food are absorbed. The jejunum and ileum further break down the food so that the body can absorb the other nutrients intended for the bloodstream.

The food goes to the large intestines. Water, electrolytes and other nutrients such as sodium and potassium are absorbed in the large intestine. When the body finishes classifying the nutrients found in the food you ate, it will transport the remaining material to the rectum. The body expels the waste through bowel movement.

Diarrhea and malabsorption occur when the stomach transports the food without digestion or partially digesting it. Since the small intestines cannot break down food without the gastric juices and other digestive enzymes from the stomach, bladder, and pancreas, they will immediately transfer the food to the large intestines.

The same goes through with the large intestines. The large intestines transfer the food to the rectum and the body expels the food through loose bowel movement.

Adjustable Gastric Banding

The first type of bariatric surgery is adjustable gastric banding or what commonly known as laparoscopic banding. This is a minimally invasive surgery. The surgeon attaches a binding in your stomach through small incisions on the upper abdomen. The banding is made of silicone and is adjustable. The most popular gastric banding is the Lap-Band under the Allergan and SAGB under the Ethicon.

The banding creates a very small pouch in the upper part of the stomach, which can only hold a ½ cup of food. This new pouch restricts the amount of food intake. You feel fuller even after eating a small portion of food.

Aside from minimal surgery invasion, another advantage of this procedure is its reversibility. You can ask to remove the banding when you have achieved your ideal weight and have the confidence to maintain your ideal weight for life.

Roux-en-Y or proximal gastric bypass

This is an irreversible surgery but many doctors recommend this to morbidly obese people because of its rapid effect. The procedure includes cutting a portion of the stomach and attaching this new pouch to the small intestine. The procedure creates a roux and a Y. It bypasses a part of the stomach. The new pouch can only hold 1 cup of food or lesser.

Other Gastric Bypass Procedures

Other procedures are gastric bypass sleeve, gastric pacing, and gastric balloon. Gastric bypass sleeve procedure involves cutting the stomach vertically and removing the fundus. The removal of the fundus shuts off ghrelin production, another type of hunger hormone. This procedure is irreversible since the operation involves removing a part of the stomach.

Gastric pacing aims to change the behavior of the digestive system, particularly the stomach. This does not require removal of any part or bypassing of the stomach. The procedure involves placement of an electrical pacing in the stomach. So far, this type of gastric surgery is still in the process of clinical study.

Gastric balloon procedure is placing a large object inside the stomach to restrict food intake. The idea of this procedure is to place the "balloon" inside the stomach for 6 months. During this period, the patient should learn to change his/her eating habits. The advantage of this procedure is its reversibility.

After 6 months, the patient undergoes another surgical procedure to remove the balloon. The disadvantage is the yo-yo effect on individuals who cannot maintain a healthy diet after the balloon removal.

The best procedure for weight loss depends on many factors. One factor you should consider is your health. You have to consult a physician about your decision to undergo gastric bypass surgery. You will take various tests such a BMI, blood test, cholesterol and other tests necessary to ensure a successful surgery. Complications might happen and you should be ready to face them.

Preparation before the Procedure

Gastric bypass surgery is a big leap on your part. There are things that you should do and prepare for. One consideration is the cost. The total cost of a procedure depends on your insurance coverage, the type of procedure and the fee of the surgeon and other health professionals involved.

Costs of the Procedure

Check your policy if it covers this kind of procedure to lessen the cost of surgery. A procedure without insurance may cost you approximately twenty thousand dollars or more. The longer you stay at the hospital the higher is your bill. One cause of staying longer in the hospital is health complications. To avoid these complications, you will undergo various lab examinations.

Aside from the cost of the procedure and the surgeon's fee, consider also the fee of other health professionals. Most likely, you might need the help of a registered dietitian. In some cases, you might need a psychologist to help you cope with the pressure of losing weight. Even if you plan your meals, consulting a dietitian is helpful.

Oftentimes, the emotional roller coaster of losing weight may take a toll on your emotional well-being. You feel like giving up or feel pressured into keeping up a diet after the surgery. A psychologist can help you unburden the stress related to a weight loss surgery. He can encourage and help you find your motivation to keep on going.

Commitment and Complications

The second factor to consider is commitment. A gastric bypass operation is a long-term commitment. The first year is somewhat easy because you see significant changes in your weight. Rapid weight loss is evident. You feel invigorated because the surgery is a success but the second year becomes a hard work.

The second year is the year of real hardship, where you need to maintain eating less food, and to continue eating at a slower pace. The question is "Are you ready for a life-long commitment, for a permanent change?"

You have to weigh the pros and cons of your decision. For the next 10 years or for the rest of your life, you can never go back to eating fast food. You will never binge. You will never eat a lot of sugary food again. You must intake lots of food supplements to replace the nutrients lost due to decreased food portion size.

Aside from these kinds of commitments, you should be ready for the health complications during your recovery. Oftentimes, you will feel nauseated and frustrated because you cannot eat the food you usually have before the procedure.

You feel heart burns because of the reflux of gastric juices in your digestive system when you eat the wrong way. Every wrong decision you make means sufferings of unimaginable pain. Read the overview of gastric bypass procedure and the related complications before making a decision.

In short, before making the decision, you should be ready for these kinds of commitment and complications. Weight loss is not an easy journey. It has always been a tough one.

You should be ready to take this journey to improve your health and well-being. The only person who can make this journey a success is you. Other professionals can help you along the way but the ultimate actor in a weight loss surgery is you.

3 - Identify Your Weight Loss Goals

Losing weight before the surgery must have been your dilemma. No diet works for you. Exercises seem a taxing activity because of your busy life. Being busy should not be a reason to stop looking for ways to lose weight.

With the rising popularity of gastric bypass surgery, you begin to contemplate that this procedure may also work for you. You ask your colleagues or friends who have undergone the same procedure and gather information about the surgery.

Your weight loss journey starts the moment you contemplate in getting a gastric bypass surgery. At this point in your journey, setting realistic goals is an essential part of succeeding in losing weight. How realistic your goals should be? What are the considerations you should make?

Remember one thing. Your weight loss journey is different from other people. On some days, you may lose a lot of weight. There will be days when you reach a plateau and do not lose weight for a few weeks or so.

Sometimes, you may even gain a little weight. If you gain a pound or two, do not fret. Your body is a complex mixture of muscles, fat, and bones. The most intelligent scientists cannot understand why people gain weight even after so many rigorous diets and exercises.

Your body is different compared to others. Never compare their milestones with yours. If it takes two to three years to achieve your weight loss goals, just let it be. Perhaps, this is how your body copes with the gastric bypass procedure. Every person has a unique way of recovering from a major surgery and of losing weight after the surgery.

Just remember to continue with what you have begun. Your weight loss journey will be fraught with so many trials and complications. Focus on your goals. Never lose hope because if you do, you will slip back to your old self, resorting to food for comfort. Always remember your goal. Focus on that. Record what you ate and what you did to achieve your goal. You need a food journal to evaluate your progress.

How do you set up your real goal? Base your decision on the average weight loss related to the surgery. If you are going to choose lap band and the average weight loss after two years is 40% of the excess of the ideal weight, set your goals on this percentage.

For example, the excess of your ideal weight is 300 pounds. Normally, you would like to lose weight as much as possible and as soon as possible. However, this does not happen all the time. To achieve your goal of losing as much as 300 pounds, do it in installments. During the first year after the surgery, your goal is to lose 120 to 150 pounds.

On the second year onwards, losing the remaining 150 to 180 pounds is your next goal. If you do not achieve your goal in the second year, maintain your new eating habit and you will see the effect in the long term.

Talk with Your Loved Ones

Before you pursue the surgery, talk to your loved ones about your decision. Discuss with them about the changes you are planning to put in place in the house, especially if you are living with a partner, your kids or parents. They should understand your plans and be ready to support you. If there is one thing you need right now, it will be their encouragement and support.

Join a Support Group

A support group can encourage you at times when you think you cannot do it anymore. The members of the group can help you endure and resist the temptation of slipping back to your old self.

You can get lots of advice from these people because they are suffering the same way you do. With a support group, you can share your pain and emotional struggles. A support group can inspire you in sharing your struggles without feeling ashamed. A support group can be the people whom you can rely on if your loved ones are skeptical about your success.

4 - Things to do Before the Procedure

Preparation for a gastric bypass surgery may take long before the actual surgery happens. You will talk to different professionals such as the surgeon, registered dietitian, your psychologist and your insurance agent. There are other things that you need to do as part of the preparation stage.

First, ask your boss if you can have a longer vacation week for the surgery and for the recovery period. If your employer does not allow you to have an extended leave, you can always seek other employment opportunities but never compromise your chance of better and healthier body.

Seek other options to earn while you are recovering from the surgery. These situations should not stop you from choosing the right surgery.

Second, start eating the way you should be eating after the surgery so you can get used to it. Drastic changes will begin after the surgery so start conditioning yourself with these changes as early as before the surgery.

Third, learn the basic diet of a gastric surgery patient. This diet significantly differs from what you used to eat.

Fourth, prepare your kitchen. Throw away or remove every junk food in your fridge, freezer, and cupboards. Donate these foods to your friends, to your neighbors or to a charity.

The last thing you want is to be reminded of those junkies and feel the craving. Remember, after the surgery, your digestive system is an entirely different one. Its functions are restricted. Your hunger hormones are reduced. You should discipline yourself and discipline starts in your kitchen.

Change your utensils into smaller versions than the regular ones. Purchase measuring cups and other pieces of equipment to measure and weigh the food you eat. This may seem a bit ridiculous but you need to measure everything you consume. If you are eating in a restaurant or dining out, remember the standard sizes for each food.

Fifth, start a journal. This journal contains your daily meal plans, the things you do while you recover from the surgery and the things you plan to do to achieve your weight loss goal. A journal can help you keep track of your progress but never include a daily monitoring of your weight.

If you want to monitor your weight, do it on a monthly or quarterly basis. Daily or weekly monitoring of the weight you lost after the surgery will just frustrate and depress you, especially if your body has a slower pace of shedding those unwanted pounds.

A food journal can help you keep track of the food that makes you nauseous or triggers vomiting. During the course of your recovery, you will likely suffer diarrhea or dumping syndrome. Jotting down everything that happens right after you eat is important. This will help you avoid the food that triggers such complications.

Before going through the procedure, make sure you have prepared everything. Make sure you are ready for all the consequences, complications and changes that will unfold in the next few months.

5 - Things to do After the Procedure

The challenge begins after the surgery. Health professionals will still care for you until your recovery is complete. However, your role has the biggest impact on the success of your gastric bypass surgery.

The tasks of maintaining a healthy body are daunting but your commitment can help achieve your goals. The journey starts with understanding how your new pouch works. It continues by learning the basic diet of post-bariatric surgery and by knowing how to handle nutrition deficiencies.

Understanding your new pouch

After the surgery, the function of your stomach is still the same except that your stomach is smaller and can only hold a ½ cup of food. Weeks or months after the surgery, your stomach's capacity increases to 1 cup of food when the swelling subsides.

Over time, your new stomach stretches but only to a limited capacity. When your stomach heals and the swelling stops, you can eat solid foods but to a maximum of one cup a meal.

Avoid overstretching your new pouch. Eat in small portions and slowly. Eat the right food and drink the right liquids. This way you can overcome the risks of dumping and vomiting.

6 - Learn the Basic Diet of Post Bariatric Surgery

The success of gastric bypass surgery depends on your commitment to learning everything you need to know so you can achieve a healthy and skinny body. This includes learning the basic diet of post-bariatric surgery. All your meal plans are based on this basic diet.

The basic diet of post gastric bypass surgery consists of 50% protein, 25% fruits and vegetables and 25% grains (or starch). The portion size is also smaller than a regular balanced meal.

The protein comprises the bulk of your diet, sharing one-half of the daily food requirements. Your protein requirement is 8 to 10 servings or approximately 60 to 80 grams of protein. The total protein requirements include the protein supplements.

Vegetables are consumed in two servings a day. The same serving sizes are required for fruits. Grains and other starchy food have a combined two servings a day while fat is required at four servings a day.

Thus, if your food intake is 1 cup for each meal, your plate should contain ½ cup of protein-rich food, ¼ cup of vegetables and fruit and ¼ cup of starch or grains.

Variety is a concept of a healthy diet especially for people who have undergone bariatric surgery. For example, milk is high in calcium but lacks iron. To get iron from food, consider consuming meat or food that is high in iron. Strawberry is a good source of Vitamin C but a carrot is high in Vitamin A.

Calories and its function in your body

Every bit of food you eat, even the junk food, provides energy. You may get many calories from eating junk foods but these foods contain empty nutrients. The wrong notion about calories is it is bad for your health and body.

Actually, the optimum level of calories fuels your body and it functions. Consumption of calories more than the recommended amount is bad for you. No matter how small the amount is, excess calories pile up and become as stored fats.

The measuring unit of energy in food is kilocalorie (kcal) or just calorie. The number of calories in a food indicates the amount of energy you can consume for a given activity or in maintaining the necessary functions of your body. Generally, the more calories consumed, the more energy you can spend on activities.

Going back to why calories are important, protein, carbohydrates, and fats provide kilocalories of energy. For every gram of protein or carbohydrates, you get 4 kcal of energy. For every gram of fat, your body expends 9 kcal of energy.

Your body requires twice the amount of energy to burn fats as compared to protein and carbohydrates. That is why fat is consumed only in moderation. Protein, carbohydrates, and fats are macronutrients that are essential in keeping the body healthy. An omission of one of these nutrients can cause nutrient deficiencies.

Protein and its part of your recovery after surgery

Protein is important in the healing process after the surgery. It helps your body heal fast and build muscles. Protein keeps your immune system working properly, maintains healthy blood and provides more energy. Protein-rich foods also contribute other nutrients such as zinc, iron, B vitamins and thiamine.

The good sources of protein are meat, milk, eggs, cheese, yogurt and other food products from animals. Although plant sources contain protein, they are low in quantity and sometimes not as high quality as the protein found in food products from animals.

Legumes, soy, tofu, and nuts are good sources of protein that is plant-based. When eating, you eat the protein-rich foods first before consuming the other foods on your plate.

The challenge in consuming protein after the surgery is that your stomach may not be able to digest it. Some bariatric patients can cope with digesting protein-rich foods without any side effect. In case your stomach cannot tolerate protein-rich foods yet, you can supplement your protein requirements with whey protein.

Protein is essential in your diet. The recommended protein intake is 15 – 20 grams every meal or a maximum daily requirement of 80 grams.

Your sources can come from the food you eat but during the recovery weeks when eating solid food is intolerable, protein supplements are enough. As your new pouch heals totally, the recommended protein sources should come from food and supplements, not just supplements alone.

Carbohydrate and its job in keeping you healthy

Carbohydrates have a bad reputation when it comes to eating healthy. Many health experts advocate that carbs should be eliminated from the diet. The truth is carbs are essential to keeping the body healthy. The important thing is to distinguish the good carbs from the bad carbs for a healthy diet.

Good carbohydrates are high in fiber, and nutrients such as Vitamin A and folate and antioxidants. Fiber does not provide nutrients but is essential in keeping a good digestive system. Sources of carbohydrates are whole grain wheat, pasta, bread and, rice, vegetables, and fruits. The daily consumption is 100 grams minimum.

Sugar is a carbohydrate. Post-gastric bypass surgery diet includes foods rich in sugars that are either naturally added or substitutes to not more than 10 grams a meal. Sugar can be a natural component of an ingredient or artificially added into the food.

Watch out for added sugars when consuming packaged food. Sugar whether natural or added should be consumed in moderation. Examples of natural sugar are fructose and lactose. Lactose is the natural sugar in milk and milk products while fructose is found in fruits.

Aside from natural sugars, you can consume sugar substitutes and sugar alcohols in moderation. Examples of sugar substitutes are Saccharin and Stevia. Sugar alcohols have a lesser amount of calories but may cause bloating or diarrhea. Examples of sugar alcohols are sorbitol and xylitol.

Fat and its role in your body

Fat is good when consumed in moderation. Your body needs fat to build cells and produce hormones. However, because of the many fad diets, people have misconceptions about fat.

Just like carbohydrates, there is a bad fat and a good fat. The good fats are essential in keeping your body healthy. Without these fats, some body parts may have difficulty performing their functions. One instance is when your body has a difficulty of supplying enough oil to your skin and hair. Without enough fats, your skin and hair become brittle and dry.

Another side effect of eliminating fats entirely from your diet is a nutrient deficiency. Some vitamins and minerals essential for body functions require fats. Fat-soluble vitamins are Vitamin A, D, E and K. Your body needs fats to break these vitamins to an absorbable level.

What are good fats and bad fats? The four major types of fats are monounsaturated, polyunsaturated, trans-fat, and saturated fats. Polyunsaturated and monounsaturated are healthy fats because these fats lower the bad cholesterol in the blood. Sources of these fats are olive oil, avocados, and some vegetable oils. Fishes are also good sources of monounsaturated and polyunsaturated fats.

Trans fat and saturated fats are bad for your health. Identifying these fats is easy. Trans-fat is present in processed food such as cookies and doughnuts while saturated fats come from animal meat sources such as chicken, beef, and pork. To avoid trans-fat totally, read labels of packaged food. Watch out for hydrogenated oils. These oils are trans-fat.

Alternatively, avoid eating processed foods. Labels may show that the processed food is trans-fat free even if the food contains less than ½ gram of trans-fat. This has something to do with government regulations and manufacturer's packaging.

Chicken meat, beef, and pork are good sources of protein. To minimize saturated fats in your diet, consume lean and organic meats. Remove visible fats when cooking meat. These fats are the real sources of saturated fats, not the lean meat. Alternately, you can eat vegetables that are rich in protein such as legumes.

Also, limit your daily intake of sodium. The daily maximum is 2,300 milligrams.

Reading Nutrition Labels

Buying packaged products such as cheese, milk and some canned goods is unavoidable. What you can do is to learn how to read nutrition labels. All packaged products have nutrition labels on them.

Look for the recommended serving size. Remember the three macronutrients when reading nutrition facts. Compare percentage daily values. The serving size describes how much calories and nutrients a serving contains.

Nutrients per serving are in percentage daily values and are measured using the standard measurement applicable to that nutrient. A percentage daily value of 5% or less is little while 15% or higher is a lot.

For example, a serving size of a packaged product gives a 440 kcal. The nutrient facts include 29% fats that composed of 21% saturated and trans fat and 36% sodium. The other nutrients facts include 18% carbohydrates with a sugar content of 6 grams and fiber of 16%. The protein content is 15 grams per serving that consists of 45% Vitamin A, 4% Vitamin C, 20% Calcium and 20% iron.

The food in the example is very high in fat since it contains 21% saturated fat. This is above the recommended 5% daily value. Avoid this type of product because it causes nausea and worsens dumping.

With regard to the sugar content, choose foods with less than 10 grams. Some people who have gastric bypass surgery report that they experience dumping when they consume more than 10 grams of sugar.

Although dumping complications vary from one bariatric patient to another, it is best to benchmark such claims. You wouldn't want to risk yourself with this complication because dumping has no cure. The only thing you can do is let it pass, which is a nightmare.

Using the food example, the sugar content is within the minimum level of 10 grams. The carbohydrate content is at an optimum level. Avoid candies, soda drinks, and other products with added sugar. Eat whole grains, vegetables, and fruits to ensure your carbohydrate intake is at the optimum level.

Protein intake is 60 to 80 grams a day. On the example, the

food contains 15 grams of protein for every 300 grams. The packaged food is at the 80-gram level but is not enough. You need to add more protein. The packaged food is very high in sodium. If you have not eaten any food with high sodium content, consuming this food is acceptable.

If in case you experience nausea or feel the need to vomit, record it in your journal. Write all the nutrition details for future reference.

How to Handle Nutrition Deficiencies

After a gastric bypass surgery, the most common side effect is nutrition deficiency. Your stomach has limited capabilities to absorb nutrients from the food you eat because of the limited amount of food intake. The most common nutrient deficiencies are Vitamin A, C, B1, and B12, iron, calcium, folate, and zinc.

The signs and symptoms may include lack of coordination and poor eyesight. It may also include slower metabolism rate, mood swings and difficulties in sustaining short and long-term memory. Malnutrition is also a common effect of bariatric surgery.

6 - LEARN THE BASIC DIET OF POST BARIATRIC SURGERY

To address nutrient deficiencies and malnutrition after a surgery, eat a balanced diet and take food supplements. A regular blood monitoring can also prevent deficiencies and malnutrition. You and your dietitian can work it out if nutrition deficiencies occur while you are recovering from the surgery.

7 - Supplementing Your Diet

There are two considerations when taking your supplement. The first consideration is taking the right supplements. The second consideration is the time of taking them.

During the first two weeks after the surgery, you need protein supplements, regardless of the type of the gastric bypass surgery. The protein powder is dissolved or is included in your liquid diet as a protein shake.

On the third week onwards, you need multivitamins, minerals, Vitamin B12, calcium and Vitamin D in addition to the protein supplements. Your dietitian may require other supplements depending on your blood tests.

The multivitamins are in chewable or liquid suspension during the recovery stage. From week 10 onwards, you can intake tablets and non-chewable medicines. By this time, your stomach is used to solid foods.

Supplements are part of your daily diet even after your stomach has healed. Taking these supplements strictly can help you keep your body healthy for life. Multivitamins and other supplements help in regulating appetite and metabolism. These can help in controlling hunger and can help in absorbing nutrients from the limited amount of food you eat.

Remember, these multivitamins are supplements and are no substitute for a healthy diet. You should prioritize eating a balanced diet and gradually lessen supplements to a small quantity or as prescribed by your dietitian or doctor.

Protein Supplements

Fifty percent of your bariatric diet comes from protein-rich foods. Sixty to eighty grams of protein is the required amount every day. For the first few weeks after surgery, reaching this required amount of protein is almost impossible.

The only way to reach the 80-gram level every day during the first few weeks is through protein supplements. You need to build muscles and retain those muscles to help in making your surgery a successful one. You know that muscles need more energy, which means you need more calories for energy. More importantly, protein helps your stomach heals and recovers fast.

Protein supplements are abundant in the market. The problem is finding a good one that tastes good, is affordable and appetizing.

You should buy protein powder that provides a maximum of 30 grams of protein, 10 grams of sugar and 5 grams of fat for each serving. Each serving can be 1 tablespoon or 1 scoop, depending on the nutrient label. Always read the nutrition facts before using a supplement in your meal.

Nowadays, a protein supplement with the highest quality is the whey protein. This is a by-product of manufacturing cheese. Since this is a by-product of milk that contains lactose, choose whey isolates if you have lactose intolerance.

Whey isolates have lower lactose compared to the standard whey powder. Watch out for protein supplements with collagen. These have low protein contents and may not be sufficient for your required daily protein intake.

You can take 1 to 2 protein shakes every day. You can also include protein supplements in your desserts. Combine these supplemental foods with the main dishes and make sure you have eaten a well-balanced diet. Never be tempted to replace natural protein sources with supplements.

Multivitamins and Other Supplements

Aside from daily protein supplements, you need to take multivitamins, too. Your surgeon and dietitian might require you to take at least one multivitamin tablet a day. If they require more than just one, follow their instructions, especially if the blood tests turn out that you are experiencing severe nutrient deficiencies.

8 - Meal Planning and its Benefits

To most people, meal planning is a time-consuming activity. If you had done meal planning before your gastric bypass surgery and failed, it could be that you are doing it the wrong way. After your surgery, meal planning should be one of your priorities before you start your day.

A 25-minute meal planning at the start of your week is not a nuisance at all if you just give it a try. Every week, schedule meal planning and make it a habit. You will be surprised to learn that it is rather easy to do. Besides, you have to master the art of meal planning so you can be sure that you are eating the most nutritious food in your new pouch.

Meal planning has many benefits. The first benefit is saving precious time in thinking what to eat and not to eat. If you spend time thinking what to eat every day, you are wasting time.

However, if you devote at least a few minutes once a week, you can use your time for other activities. You do not need to rush to the grocery to buy certain ingredients. You do not need to thaw an ingredient for the last minute cooking.

The second benefit is adding variety to your meals. List

every meal that you usually cook for a week. You might be surprised to find out that in a week you are cooking the same meal all over again. With meal planning, you can introduce a new recipe in your meal. You can apply the principle of variety when preparing meals, or increase your chance of getting the necessary food nutrients that your body needs.

The third benefit is saving money. When you are done planning your meal for at least two weeks, you can list all the items you need to buy in the grocery. Perhaps, you can even find a bulk discount for buying bulk items or bargain items. You do not need to buy items that you do not use. No more impulsive buying, ever again. You can go to the grocery once a week and save time and fuel expense.

The fourth benefit is enjoying a stress-free meal. After the surgery, you have a few days off but you have to go back to your work soon. With meal planning, you do not have to worry what to prepare because you already have prepared your food for the week. Just get the food from your fridge, cook it or place it in a microwave and wait for your food while you relax and read your favorite book or watch the latest news.

The fifth benefit is enjoying the food you love to eat except that the ingredients are more nutritious. For example, your favorite is burger and fries. You do not need to forgo these foods. To make it healthier and friendlier to your new pouch than the usual burger and fries, try buying burger patties with less fat.

You can even make a healthier version of the patty such as making it with veggies as substitute ingredients. Instead of cooking it in oil, try using a nonstick pan to fry the patty. Alternatively, grill the patty for a different taste. For the bun, use whole grain. For the fries, instead of deep-frying, try baking it with olive oil, pepper, and salt as seasonings.

Meal planning is easy and fun. You can still eat your favorite food without compromising your healthy diet. You can use substitutes so you can still eat what you usually eat with a few modifications.

With meal planning, you can change your eating habits one step at a time. You can change your lifestyle and make your gastric bypass surgery a successful one.

Stock Your Kitchen with Nutritious Ingredients

Fruits, vegetables, meat, and grains should be part of your kitchen. Aside from these essential ingredients for cooking, buy herbs and spices.

Herbs are dried leaves and stems of plants. Examples of herbs are basil, bay leaves, oregano, coriander and lemongrass. Spices are dried seeds and bark of a plant. Examples of spices are pepper, garlic, onion, and paprika. Herbs and spices can help you spice up an ordinary food. These ingredients are also rich in vitamins and minerals that you need to combat nutrient deficiency.

Aside from these ingredients, nutritious oil for cooking is also an important addition to your kitchen. Olive oil, canola oil, and sesame oil are better alternatives than using lard or ordinary vegetable oil. Extracts should also be part of your cooking ingredients. Examples of extracts are lemon, vanilla, and almond extracts. You can use these extracts to flavor up baked goodies, drinks, and other main dishes.

Conclusion

A gastric bypass surgery entails major changes in your life. These changes include learning how to forgo your bad eating habits and changing your bad eating habits into healthier ones. You can start implementing these changes by stocking your kitchen with fruits and vegetables and by learning the basic diet of post-bariatric surgery.

9 - Coping with Complications and Other Health Issues

Like any other major surgeries, you might experience complications and other health issues. No matter how strict you are with your diet and how good you are at following orders from your surgeon and physician, you might still encounter complications more than once.

Stomach Pain, Nausea, and Vomiting

These are common sicknesses during the recovery phase. This might be due to your body's reaction to the anesthesia wearing off and your body's way of coping with your new pouch. After recovery, these might be caused by several reasons such as eating the wrong food in the wrong way.

Other reasons may include eating and drinking at the same time, eating too fast, swallowing without chewing the food thoroughly, drinking carbonated drinks and dehydration.

The risks of continued vomiting due to your carelessness may include obstruction in the opening of your stomach due to swelling, hernia and tearing apart of the incisions in your stomach and your abdomen.

Dehydration and nutrient deficiency may also be a risk if your vomiting continues. When vomiting persists even after avoiding the food, you should not eat and after taking all the precautionary measures, visit your doctor to determine what is causing it.

To avoid nausea and vomiting, eat slowly and chew your food thoroughly. Stop drinking carbonated drinks. Instead, drink lots of water and non-sugary liquids. Even if you have recovered from the surgery, it is best to become steadfast in your weight loss goals.

Constipation

Anesthesia and the pain medications you are taking while in the hospital may cause constipation. To deal with constipation, drink lots of liquid to help your intestines flush out the toxins in your body.

Move a lot. If constipation persists after hospitalization, insufficient drinking of fluids is a possible cause. It is normal to experience constipation during the recovery stage after the surgery because of the restricted intake of fiber.

Follow the recommended daily liquid intake. By the end of week 9, you should be drinking 6 to 8 glasses of water to keep you hydrated and to help your intestines do their job. You may use suppositories and stool softeners to help you alleviate constipation. Before using these stool softeners, consult your surgeon first.

By week 10 and onwards, you can include fresh fruits and cooked vegetables to complete your daily requirements of fiber. Consumption of fiber can help alleviate constipation.

Diarrhea

This is another complaint of most bariatric surgery patients. Reasons may include an inability of the stomach to absorbed fat, sugar substitutes, lactose intolerance and certain food intolerance. If you are experiencing 4 – 5 loose bowels in a day, visit your surgeon to see what is causing your diarrhea.

Do not attempt to cure your diarrhea by taking medicines. Remember, you have a digestive tract with limited capabilities. The standard medicines for curing diarrhea may not be applicable to you anymore. There is one thing you can do, though. Do not stop drinking fluids to compensate for the lost liquid in your body.

Dehydration

It can be caused by severe vomiting or insufficient drinking of liquids. Dehydration is normal a day or two after a gastric bypass surgery due to the difficulty of tolerating liquid. Common symptoms include parched lips, dry skin and eyes, dizziness, irritability and dark urine.

Drink lots of liquid. If you cannot tolerate plain water, spice it up with flavor. Just remember to drink sugar-free or low-calorie juice. You may also slurp a no-sugar ice-pop as desired. Use the same container to track your liquid intake. Fresh fruit juices are okay as long as they are diluted with water. Your juice drink should be half fruit juice and half plain water.

After day three of your surgery, you should be able to tolerate most types of liquid. If you cannot tolerate drinking liquids by this time, consult your surgeon.

Food Intolerance

After the surgery, food intolerance is normal because of the altered state of your stomach. Common symptoms include a feeling of stuffiness in your stomach as if foods are trapped in the opening of your stomach or an incessant pain that does not go away even after a few hours after eating. The best thing you can do is to record such feelings of pain whenever you eat and discuss these with your surgeon.

Foods such as bread, pasta, milk and milk products, and red meat might cause food intolerance. You should avoid eating these foods during the first 9 weeks. If you cannot help but experiment, just remember to record any incidence of food intolerance in your journal.

Lactose Intolerance

This could happen during the first 9 weeks. You may experience lactose intolerance after the surgery. This is due to the restricted ability of the stomach to produce gastric juices necessary to digest lactose.

If you suddenly develop intolerance to milk and milk

products, stop drinking them. Common symptoms may include bloating, stomach pain and diarrhea. If you are worried about calcium deficiency, you can always take supplements.

Dumping Syndrome

This is common to all types of gastric bypass surgeries. This happens when food moves fast from the stomach to the small intestines. Dumping syndrome is characterized by nausea, abdominal cramps, cold sweats, weakness, explosive diarrhea, fast heartbeat, dizziness and upset stomach. Two or three of these symptoms indicate you are suffering the feared dumping syndrome.

Food with high fat and high sugar content can cause dumping. Dumping syndrome may occur immediately after eating, as immediately as 15-30 minutes or 2-4 hours after eating. Dumping can last for hours depending on the amount of sugary or fatty foods you have eaten. There is no cure for dumping or no medicine to alleviate the pain. The only thing you can do is to lie down and wait for it to pass.

Not everyone with bypassed stomach experiences dumping.

Some may experience worse dumping syndrome than others are. Those who are unlucky, the dumping syndrome can become a chronic condition for the rest of their lives. Other people may only experience it temporarily.

They may also get the same reaction if they eat certain foods. Dumping syndrome may occur less as time passes since you already have a better understanding of how your new stomach works. You already know which food brings such occurrences.

Although every person's experience with dumping is unique, you can minimize dumping syndrome by avoiding foods with more than 10 grams of sugar such as chocolate, sports drink, frozen fruit with heavy syrup, and undiluted fruit juices.

Avoid consuming fatty foods such as hot dogs, French fries, and deep-fried foods. Remember the 5% to 15% daily values. If a food contains more than 15% of fats, it is considered as very high in fats.

On week 10 onwards, try eating more foods rich in fiber. Eat frequent small meals, instead of eating big meals for breakfast, lunch, and dinner. Include foods with complex carbohydrates and increase intake of food rich in protein and supplements.

Reactive Hypoglycemia

Reactive hypoglycemia happens after eating wherein your body's sugar level drops below the ideal level. The ideal blood sugar level is 4 mmol/L. Even if you do not have diabetes prior to your surgery, you may still experience this kind of complication.

When food with high sugar or fat content goes to the small intestine without being broken down properly, the pancreas produces more insulin to digest the food. As a result, your sugar level drops below the minimum. Symptoms may include hunger, clammy and cold skin, dizziness or shakiness, feeling of confusion and nervousness.

If you suspect reactive hypoglycemia, take your blood sugar level with a blood glucose meter. If the results are below the minimum, drink fast-acting sugar, approximately 15 grams. Examples of fast acting sugars are dextrose tablets, honey, and sugar dissolved in water. Wait for 15 minutes before checking your blood sugar.

If the level remains below the minimum, repeat drinking fast-acting sugar and check after 15 minutes. Alternatively, eat a small snack with protein and carbohydrates. This snack can consist of Greek yogurt with fresh fruits, peanut butter, and apple.

Do not eat foods with high sugar such as candies and cakes to elevate the level of your sugar. These foods have different sugar contents and may have an adverse effect on your blood sugar. Remember, reactive hypoglycemia happens because your stomach did not churn the food high in sugar and fat.

You can prevent hypoglycemia from happening. Do not skip meals and eat your meals on time. Do not drink alcohol and do not eat food with high sugar content and fat. As always, balanced diet is important.

Bloating

Gas in your stomach is normal. This happens when you "swallow" gas while eating and drinking. Soda drinks can also cause gas to accumulate in your stomach. This results in bloating.

This is painful and may overstretch your new stomach. You can prevent gas or bloating by eating slowly. Do not use a straw while sipping liquids. Avoid chewing gums. Remember to record in your food journal the food that causes bloating.

Hair Loss

Hair loss can be related either to poor nutrition or to the surgery. If hair loss happens right after the surgery, it is your body's response to the stress of undergoing the procedure. If it happens weeks after the surgery, the likely cause is nutrient deficiency such as iron or zinc deficiency. Hair loss may also be due to low protein intake.

Hair loss related to the surgery is not preventable. Besides, your hair will grow back once you have recovered. Hair loss due to nutrient deficiency is manageable. To prevent hair loss due to poor nutrition, make sure to eat foods rich in iron and zinc. Take protein supplements religiously.

Conclusion

Complications may vary from one person to another. You may experience worse complications compared to others. In some days, you feel fine. In other days, you feel worse than eating a single meal is a chore. Whatever complications you experience after your surgery, always consult your doctor about it.

Do not forget to write any symptom or complication you experience after drinking a certain liquid or eating a specific food. One way of keeping complications at bay is to become aware of what might happen and what will happen if you eat this and drink that. The only way to monitor is to keep a journal.

Complications are normal to some extent. If complications do not go away after three days, consult with your doctor right away.

10 - Week 1 to 2 after Surgery – Liquid Diet

The first few weeks after the surgery may be difficult since your food and liquid intake are restricted. After the surgery, you have to introduce food gradually to your new digestive system. While you are in the hospital for two to three days, or more depending on the type of the surgery done to you, your diet includes clear liquid and nothing else.

Day 1 and 2 after the surgery

It is a bit weird to drink liquids for breakfast, snacks, lunch, or dinner but it is the only "food" your stomach can tolerate as it heals. Clear liquid diet may include water, broth with different flavors, fruit juice diluted with water and no sugar added to it.

This type of diet will last for two days or up to a week, depending on your stomach's tolerance for new foods. Even if you are on IV fluid while in the hospital, you need to sip liquids to know if your stomach is working fine. During the clear liquid diet, try sipping at least 30 ml every 15 minutes on the first day and at least 60 ml of water every thirty minutes on the second day.

Oranges, lemon, strawberries, and blueberries are the examples of fruits that you can soak in the water to give flavor to your water. However, orange juices are not allowed during the first two weeks of your recovery.

Sample Clear Liquid Diet

When preparing broth for your liquid diet, make sure you remove the fats from the beef. Skin from organic chicken is okay to include when boiling it. Your new pouch cannot tolerate fatty foods yet.

You can add spices and herbs to spice the flavor of your liquid diet but limit it. You can add mint leaves in your tea or juice but do not eat the leaves. You can consume coffee and tea since these are considered clear liquids once diluted with water.

For breakfast:

- Mango, Apple, or Pineapple Juice diluted in water

- Broth (chicken or beef flavor)

- Gelatin without sugar

- Decaffeinated coffee

Snack

- No sugar clear liquid supplement

Lunch

- Beef broth

- Sugar-free gelatin

- Tea, no sugar with a few mint leaves for flavor

- No sugar popsicles

Snack

- No sugar clear liquid supplement

Dinner

- Broth (chicken, beef or pork)

- Flavored water no sugar

- No sugar popsicles

- Gelatin without sugar

Snack

- No sugar clear liquid supplement

On the second day, you can rearrange the order of this menu. It is a bit boring but you have to tolerate this diet. Besides, it only lasts for a few weeks or so until you can introduce solid foods to your diet. You can drink the liquids warm or cold, depending on your stomach tolerance.

Week 1 to Week 2 after the Surgery

Your first week starts after your doctor discharges you from the hospital. On the third day, assuming you stayed in the hospital for two days, try introducing full liquids to your clear liquid diet. Full liquid diet includes all the clear liquid diet in the first two days after surgery and full liquids.

A full liquid diet may include skimmed milk with 1% fat, hot dark chocolate without sugar, soya milk, buttermilk, low-fat pureed soups, thoroughly cooked cereals with a soupy consistency, juices diluted with water, no sugar puddings or custard, light yogurt without sugar and protein shakes.

You can include potatoes pureed in soupy consistency. Other vegetables that you can make into pureed soups include tomato, squash, carrots and other starchy vegetables that can be mashed and turned into pureed soup.

Full liquid diet lasts for two weeks. During these weeks, start taking your protein supplements. Protein helps your stomach heals fast. You can also start taking chewable vitamins and mineral supplements. Follow the doses your dietitian recommended you to take.

Remember to drink at least 48 ounces of liquid every day. Half of the required liquid intake daily may come from the clear liquid diet and the other half may come from full liquid diet. Sip the liquids and do not gulp. Take at least 20 minutes to finish a meal even if it is liquid.

If you start vomiting or nauseated after introducing full liquid diet, you can revert back to clear liquid for 24 hours. Then, proceed with full liquid diet wherein 70% consisted of clear liquid diet.

Gradually, change the ratio from 70% clear liquid and 30% full liquid to 50% clear liquid and 50% full liquid, until your stomach can tolerate full liquid. By the end of the second week, you should be able to introduce pureed diet. Otherwise, visit your doctor if you cannot tolerate pureed diet.

Examples of Full Liquid Diet

Here is an example of full liquid diet plan:

Breakfast

- Prepare oatmeal cooked in a ¼ cup of milk with 1 tablespoon of whey protein.

- Plain yogurt in small container with no sugar and low -fat content

Morning Snack

- 1 cup of protein shake

Lunch

- ¼ cup of Applesauce

- ¼ cup of Mushroom Soup with 1 tablespoon of whey protein

Afternoon snack

- ½ cup of protein shake

Dinner

- ¼ cup of cottage cheese, no fat

- Plain yogurt with 1 tablespoon of whey protein

Tips to Remember

Do not forget to drink water or any of the clear liquid diet mentioned earlier in between meals. You can also add chicken or beef broth in your meals. For breakfast, you can sip a ½ cup of chicken broth. On lunch, you can drink diluted juice drink. For meals with milk, use no fat to 1% fat or skim milk. Use salt sparingly, too.

Here is another example plan of a full liquid diet:

Breakfast

- Fruit Shake

- Plain yogurt

Snack

- Protein Shake

Lunch

- ¼ cup cottage cheese, no fat or low-fat

- ¼ cup of plain yogurt

- Diluted tomato juice

Snack

- Protein Shake

Dinner

- Chicken soup

- ¼ cup of applesauce

Snack

- Protein shake

After surgery, you might experience a temporary case of lactose intolerance. You can follow a lactose-free liquid diet. Here is an example of a lactose-free diet meal plan:

Breakfast

- Chai protein shake

Snack

- Oatmeal cooked in 1 cup of soy milk, no sugar or lactose-free milk

Lunch

- Potato soup with 1 tablespoon of protein powder (1/2 cup)

- ¼ cup of diluted tomato juice

Snack

- Protein shake

Dinner

- Vegetable soup with 1 tablespoon of protein powder (1/2 cup)

- Applesauce measuring ¼ cup

Snack

- ¼ cup of Cream of Wheat

As you can see, the goal of a liquid diet is to eat meals and drink liquids in small portion, frequently. Follow this example so you can gradually prepare your stomach for the next stage, eating pureed diet.

11 - Simple Recipes for Applesauce, Fruit Shakes, and Protein Shakes

The above examples of the liquid diet include applesauce, protein shakes and fruit shakes. You can include these meals in planning your meals even after week 10. Here are the sample recipes for these meals.

Applesauce

This recipe calls for:

- Apples with approximate total weight of 4 pounds (around 10 apples)

- Lemon zest, 4 strips

- Lemon juice to taste (approx. 3-4 tablespoons)

- Cinnamon stick

- Sugar, dark brown, ¼ cup

- Sugar, white, ¼ cup

- Water (1 cup)

- Salt (1/2 teaspoon)

Procedure for cooking:

Peel, remove seeds and quarter the apples. Boil quartered apples in 1 cup of water with the lemon, sugar, salt, and cinnamon for 20 to 30 minutes or until apples are cooked and very tender. Remove cinnamon stick and lemon peel. Mash the apples for a coarse applesauce. Blend if you want a smoother, pureed consistency.

Tips to remember

Since you are a gastric bypass patient, you can use a sugar substitute such as honey. Alternately, cut to half the amount of sugar or remove the sugar. Applesauce is a good pair for yogurt and cottage cheese. Later on, you can pair it with savory dishes when you are eating more solid foods. Freeze the applesauce for later use. The recipe yields 1 1/2 to 2 quarts or approximately 8 cups.

Fruit Shake or Protein Shake

- Protein powder (1 scoop)

- Skim milk or low-fat milk or soy milk for a lactose-free diet (1 cup)

- Vanilla extract (1 teaspoon)

- Strawberry flavored no sugar drink crystals (1/2 packet)

- Crushed ice (1/2 cup)

Procedure for preparation:

Blend all the ingredients until smooth. For an alternative, use fresh strawberry. However, make sure that the pureed strawberry has no lumps and is blended very well. You can use other fruits for your protein shakes such as banana or apple. You can also use Greek yogurt or plain yogurt instead of milk.

Chai Protein Shake

This shake calls for:

- Protein powder, vanilla flavor (1 scoop)

- Chai tea, brewed (1/3 cup)

- Soy milk, no sugar (alternative: lactose-free milk) (1/3 cup)

- Pumpkin pie spice (1/4 teaspoon)

- Ice cubes (2 pieces)

- Peach (if fresh, ½ of the fruit; if frozen, 4 slices)

Procedure:

- Blend all ingredients until very smooth. You may add more ice cubes if you like.

Tips to Remember

If you do not want to prepare your protein shakes, you can buy pre-made shakes in the grocery. You should look for pre-made protein shakes that have 15 to 40 grams of protein and less than 5 grams of carbohydrates with fiber content already subtracted. For example, a protein shake contains 5 grams of carbohydrates, with 3 grams of dietary fiber. The carbohydrate content is 2 grams.

12 - Week 3 to 4 after the Surgery – Pureed Diet

On the third week until the fourth week after your surgery, you can introduce pureed or smoothie diet. Anything that is blended and turned into pureed food can be part of this diet. Foods may include blended fruits, meats, starchy vegetables, and even eggs. As long as no sugar is added to the smoothie and fat is kept to 1% for milk add-ons, you can include it in your smoothie diet.

You can only eat one-fourth cup of the smoothie food. Don't be disappointed. The most important thing is taking the slow way of healing your new pouch. You do not need to rush. Eventually, you will be enjoying other solid foods later.

You still have to maintain at least 1 liter of liquid intake, including clear and full liquids. You have to stay hydrated so that you don't experience constipation during these weeks of recovery. Do not forget to take your protein supplements and vitamins for a faster recovery and to avoid nutrient deficiency.

Example of Pureed Diet

Breakfast

- Cream of wheat (1/4 cup) with skimmed milk (4 tablespoons)

- Pureed fruit (2 tablespoons)

Snack

- Protein Shake (1 cup)

Lunch

- Poached small egg (1 piece)

- Melba toast (1 or 2 pieces)

Snack

- Protein Shake or Plain Yogurt (1 cup)

Dinner

- Pureed meat or mashed fish (4 tablespoons)

- Mashed potato with 1 tablespoon of protein powder (3 tablespoons)

- Mashed or pureed carrots (2 tablespoons)

Evening Snack

- Protein shake (1 cup)

How to Puree Food

You can puree fruits, vegetables, and meats. Fruits and vegetables are the easiest and meat is the hardest to puree. You can keep pureed fruits and vegetables for 8 months, provided they are frozen. Pureed meat and fish can only last for 10 weeks if frozen. However, to avoid contamination, eat pureed foods immediately or store them up to 2 weeks.

For 1/3 to 1/2 cup of cooked fruits, you need 2 teaspoons or 10 ml of liquid. Blending time is 15 – 45 seconds. This serving yields 1/3 to ½ cup of pureed fruits. A ¾ cup of cooked vegetables requires 3 teaspoons of liquid and yields 1/3 to ½ cup of pureed vegetables. Blending time is 1 – 2 minutes.

A ½ cup of cooked meat requires 4 tablespoons of liquid and yields 1/3 to ½ cup of pureed meat. Blending time depends on the consistency you want or until meat is smooth and no meaty fiber is evident.

For a thicker consistency, you can add starchy and mashed food such as potato, sweet potato or squash. For a thinner consistency, add milk, water for pureeing fruits or broth if you are blending vegetables and meat.

How to Prepare Pureed Meat

It is a bit unbecoming to blend meat for your meals but you have to tolerate it. This is a way of introducing solid food, despite its blended state, to your stomach. Do not worry. This diet only lasts for 2 weeks. There are times that your doctor may advise you to introduce soft diet even before your fourth week ends.

Pureed Beef

This recipe calls for:

- Lean beef, cut into 1-inch cube (225 grams)

- Water (1 cup)

- Salt and pepper to taste

Procedure for Pureeing:

Boil the beef cubes in a saucepan for 30 minutes or until tender. Let it cool after cooking and then freeze it in the refrigerator. Reserve the broth for blending. After freezing the beef, blend it with the broth until smooth. Add salt and pepper to taste. Place it in a sealed container, leaving a few inches space as room for expansion. Label your beef puree.

Pureed chicken or turkey

This recipe calls for:

- 500 g of chicken or turkey with skin and bone intact

- 2 cups of water

- ½ teaspoon of thyme (or a few leaves of lemongrass)

- Salt and pepper to taste

Procedure for Pureeing:

Cook meat in a saucepan with the leaves of lemongrass until chicken or turkey meat separates easily from the bone. Let it cool. Disregard lemongrass. Cut into pieces and blend with the broth, thyme, salt, and pepper. Properly label your pureed chicken.

You can also add vegetables and spices when cooking the meat. Blend the meat with the vegetables with a flavorful pureed chicken or beef.

Legumes Puree

Legumes are packed with vitamins, minerals, and protein. These can be protein substitute if you are following a vegetarian diet. This recipe calls for:

- 1 cup of legumes of your choice

- 8 cups of water

- ½ teaspoon cumin powder

- Salt and pepper to taste

Procedure for pureeing:

Boil 1 cup of legumes in a saucepan with 3 cups of water for 2 minutes. Soak the legumes overnight. Drain the following morning. Add 5 cups of water and cook for 45 minutes to 1 hour. You can also use a pressure cooker to reduce the time of cooking. Remove from heat and let it cool. Blend the legumes with ¾ cups of the vegetable broth. Place in a container and label it. Freeze for later use.

You can use canned legumes for this recipe. Just blend and eat. Watch out for high-sodium content and always read the nutrient labels.

13 - Week 5 to 9 after the surgery – Soft diet

On the fifth until the ninth week, introduce soft foods in your diet. The key is to introduce gradually the solid foods into your existing diet. If your stomach cannot tolerate soft foods, go back to the pureed diet for a few days then start introducing soft food again.

This takes a trial and error to know what your stomach can or cannot tolerate. Just remember to write everything in your journal so that you know which foods to avoid and which foods to eat.

This is the time to start thinking what foods are nutritious to consume. You can now replace or reduce the number of the supplements you are taking with those nutritious foods. This is the week to start eating a balanced diet albeit a slow one.

The food that you can eat in this phase of your recovery can include ground meat to ground fish, vegetables cooked thoroughly and fruits. You can still include smoothies. Always remember to drink lots of water throughout the day.

Examples of Soft Diet

Day 1 – 80 grams of protein

Breakfast

- Fruits of your choice, fresh or canned (1/4 cup)

- Ricotta cheese (1/4 cup)

- Bran flakes with a sprinkle of cinnamon powder (1 tablespoon)

Snack – Morning

- Protein Fruit Shake

Lunch

- String Cheese (1 piece)

- Bean soup (1/2 cup)

- Melba toast (1 piece)

- Snack – Afternoon

- Yogurt or protein shake

Dinner

- Chicken soup (2 ounces)

- Thoroughly cooked vegetables (2 tablespoons)

- Mashed potato or carrots (1/4 cup)

Snack – Evening

- Tuna pita (1/4 cup tuna, light mayo, and pita bread)

- Protein Shake

Take note: Pita bread must be whole wheat and limit your mayo to 2 tablespoons.

Day 2 – 65 grams of protein

Breakfast

- Omelet using 1 egg, 2 tablespoons of diced ham (or cooked meat) and 1 tablespoon shredded cheese, low-fat

Snack – morning

- None (or plain yogurt)

Lunch

- Ground beef with gravy, low-fat

- Well-cooked broccoli (or any vegetable of your choice)

- Fruit cocktail in its own juice

Snack – afternoon

- Pudding or protein shakes (if protein requirement is not met)

Dinner

- Baked fish (3 ounces)

- Beans, thoroughly cooked (1/4 cup)

- Mashed potatoes (1/4 cup)

Snack – evening

- Milk, low-fat (1 cup)

14 - Beyond Week 10 – the New and Healthier You

If you think week 1 to 9 is the hardest, think again. The most difficult part of a gastric bypass recovery is week 10 onwards. By this time, your stomach has healed and you can tolerate most of the solid foods. The urge to try and eat the foods you usually eat before the surgery becomes stronger. You feel confident that you can make the right decisions when it comes to eating healthy.

When you think you are doing it right, your decision fails you. If it happens to you, do not despair. You make mistakes. Every one commits them. Learn from your mistakes to strive in achieving a better and healthier you.

Change in lifestyle is the key to the success of a gastric bypass procedure. This includes changing the food you eat, portion sizes, the type of food, exercise habits and the way you are chewing your food. Post gastric bypass diet is a transition from a liquid diet to soft solid food. It includes the transition from eating junk foods to eating nutritious foods.

Make eating healthy a lifelong commitment. You need to

understand the different components of what consists of a nutritious food.

Post gastric bypass diet is an entirely different diet because you need to eat smaller portion sizes of the food than you used to eat. It involves chewing your food thoroughly to make digestion easier for your smaller stomach. Since serving sizes are smaller, your stomach and body absorb fewer nutrients than before the procedure. This requires a lifelong intake of vitamins and other supplements.

Learning the Different Cooking Methods

Cooking is an art but it also involves a systematic method of food preparation. Cooks invented recipes so other people can cook the same way they do. Shortcuts and experimentation are acceptable when you are cooking. However, when you want the same result as that of the recipe, you should follow the exact ingredients and instructions.

Every recipe involves different cooking methods. Each method yields different cooked foods. In a recipe, you might read or hear the words broil, braise and sauté. If you are a beginner in cooking, these words may seem similar but these cooking methods are different.

The recommended cooking method for the meat of land animals is dry cooking. Dry cooking methods include grilling, sautéing, roasting, broiling, baking and rotisserie cooking.

Dry cooking retains moisture in the meat. This cooking method is recommended during the first three months after the surgery when food tolerance is very low. This cooking method makes the meat and fish easier to chew, swallow and digest.

The most common dry cooking is sautéing because of its short preparation time. The method of sautéing is cooking food in a pan with a minimum amount of cooking oil. Preheating is a requirement before putting oil and before cooking the food.

This method is quick and easy. It takes only 7 minutes and requires slicing the meat into thin strips. While sautéing, do not walk away from the stove. If you walk away for a few minutes, you might burn the food.

Rotisserie cooking is rotating the food over dry heat while

cooking. Grilling is cooking food with heat from below with a charcoal or flame. Roasting is cooking food in a dry heat using fat or cooking oil. Broiling is cooking food with heat from above the food. Grilling, roasting, and broiling are slow-cooking dry methods.

These methods take a minimum of one hour of preparation time. You can use these methods if preparing a weekend party or gathering where you have enough time to prepare the foods.

The second cooking method is moist cooking. This method involves boiling, deep-frying, pan-frying, stewing, poaching, and braising. Stewing is cooking food cut into small pieces in a pot with liquid.

The food is cooked on a low flame with the lid on the pot. Braising is similar to stewing except that food is cooked with a minimal amount of liquid in an oven. Boiling is cooking the food in liquid under extreme heat. Poaching is cooking food at a simmer point.

Food Safety is Important

There are times that you cannot eat everything on your plate. You do not need to fill your stomach to a brim and that you should listen to your fullness signals. To avoid wasting food, you can preserve leftovers for later consumption. When you think you cannot eat everything on your plate, place the leftover in a sealed container and freeze the food.

Do not let the food sit for more than fifteen minutes or exposed to avoid contamination or germs getting on the food. For cooked food, consume the leftover within 24 hours to 3 days. Label your container when the leftover food is placed in the fridge so you can track the date and know how many days or hours have passed since the cooking.

Measure Everything

You have learned throughout this book that you should weigh your food and measure your liquids. The thing is how do you measure food?

There are different types of ounces in measuring weight and

volume. Fluid ounces are used to measure all kinds of liquid that literally pours such as water, broth, vinegar or milk.

In some recipes, ounces are used to measure weight but this measurement is not the same as fluid ounces. If you are not familiar with the English metric, you can always convert the measuring unit into the standard unit of measurement.

For example, you see a recipe that requires 3 ounces of milk. This means you should use fluid ounces and use a measuring cup for liquids. If you see an ingredient indicating 3 ounces of chicken, you should use weighing tools to measure solid food in ounces. Other recipes use the standard metric system, which is easier since most kitchen measuring tools are in standard metric.

To make measuring easier and faster, buy two sets of measuring cups and spoons, one for measuring liquid and one for measuring dry and solid food. You should also have a small weighing scale to measure food in grams.

In measuring flour, sift first before measuring. Flour tends to compact when packed in the bag. Sifting removes the compactness of the flour. The level measurement means you have to remove the excess ingredients by leveling the measured food with a measuring cup. You can do this using a knife or a spoon to level the ingredient with the cup.

The packed measurement means you have to press down the ingredients into the measuring cup. The unpacked measurement means you just scoop an ingredient and let it as is. Food with smaller cuts tends to have more contents than with food cut into bigger cuts.

Conclusion

Learn to cook so you can choose the ingredients in your food. You can substitute unhealthy ingredients with healthy ones. You may not learn cooking immediately but making the effort to learn how to cook will pay off.

To create a daily meal plan, choose 2-3 servings of protein-rich food, 2 servings of fruits and vegetables and 2 servings of grains or starchy food for every meal.

15 - Simple Breakfast Ideas

Breakfast is the most important meal of the day. So, never skip one. Eat a hearty meal to start your day. Here are sample breakfast ideas you can include in your daily meal plan. Just remember the basics, 50% protein, 25% fruit and vegetables and 25% grains or starchy food.

Toast and Fruit

- A slice of toast with 1 tablespoon of peanut butter

- Scrambled eggs with shrimp

- Small banana

- Berry Parfait

Start your day with a low-fat no-sugar yogurt (1/2 cup). Add cereal (1/4 cup) and 3 slices of strawberries.

Savory Crackers

- Ryvita crackers (2 pieces) or English muffin (1/2)

- Tomato (1 slice)

- Cottage cheese (1/4 cup)

- Pepper

- Egg Wrap

Sauté 1 slice of ham (diced) and 2 slices of tomato (diced). Add one egg. Cook for 1 minute. Roll egg scramble in a whole wheat tortilla wrap. Eat half of the egg wrap and refrigerate the remaining half for tomorrow.

Fruity Wrap

Use a whole wheat tortilla wrap. Spread almond butter (2 tablespoons). Top it with applesauce (1/4 cup) and a pinch of cinnamon. Eat half of the roll and refrigerate the rest. Consume the other half for tomorrow.

16 - Easy Lunch Choices

With your busy life, forgetting lunch is a common occurrence. Stop this nasty habit and start preparing your lunch beforehand. You can bring with you a hearty sandwich or tortilla wrap for a quick but satisfying lunch. If you are up early or have time to prepare food in the evening, you can cook your food for lunch, freeze it and then just heat it when you're ready to eat lunch.

Cheesy Quesadilla

Use 1 small tortilla wrap, whole wheat. Top it with tomato (2 slices), spinach leaves without stem (6 pieces) and shredded fat-free cheddar cheese (1/4 cup). Fold the tortilla wrap in half. Bake the wrap in the microwave oven until the cheese melts.

Sandwiches for Lunch

Lightly spread a toasted English muffin with 1 teaspoon of low-fat mayonnaise. Top ½ of it with light cow cheese and smoked salmon (1/4 cup), capers (3 pieces), and chopped spring mix salad (1/2 cup). Alternately, use hummus (1/4 cup) and 3 slices of cucumber. Sprinkle salt and pepper to taste.

17 - Fast and Easy Dinner Options

Most of the times, eating dinner seems a chore. No matter how tired you are, fix yourself a quick dinner. Your stomach needs food to grind even if it is so small. It still releases hunger hormones and it needs something to grind on while you sleep.

Burger and fries

Who says you cannot enjoy your favorite burger and fries? You still can as long as you use a low-fat burger or a vegetarian patty. You can make the patty when you are not busy and have time to prepare it. Use a whole wheat burger bun (small) and top it with a ½ burger patty and spring mix salad. Skip the mayo. If you cannot skip it, use light mayonnaise. Oven-bake 4 fries to complete your dinner.

Breaded Chicken

Thaw 2 ounces of chicken, sliced into small cubes. Coat the chicken with crushed bran buds. Bake until the chicken is cooked. Serve it with tomato and cucumber (1/2 cup). For extra flavor, toss the tomato and cucumber salad with balsamic vinegar.

Chili

Prepare a ½ cup of salad mixed greens and chili (1/2 cup). Add sour cream in low-fat (1 tablespoon) and shredded cheese. Limit cheese to a sprinkle.

Stir-fry Seafood

Stir-fry shrimp (4 pieces) and vegetables (1/2 cup) in a teaspoon of canola oil. You can add peppers and mushrooms. Top the stir-fried seafood in couscous (1/4 cup) and a dash of soy sauce in reduced sodium content.

Sample Homemade Burger Recipe

If you are craving for burger and fries, use this recipe to make your burger patties. Store leftover patties and use them on other occasions. Preparation time is 10 minutes. This recipe yields 4 servings (4 ounces for each patty).

This recipe calls for:

- Turkey breast (1 pound, ground)

- Ginger root, peeled, chopped (1 teaspoon)

- Garlic, chopped (2 teaspoons)

- Sesame oil (1 teaspoon)

- Fresh mushrooms, chopped (1/2 cup)

- Onion powder (1 teaspoon)

- Black pepper (1/4 teaspoon)

- Soy sauce (1 tablespoon, low sodium content)

Procedure:

Preheat oven (350 degrees). Spray baking sheet with non-stick cooking spray. Combine all ingredients in a bowl. Form 4 patties and place them on the baking sheet. Bake the patties for a total of 15 minutes. Bake each side for 7 ½ minutes. Alternately, you can grill the patties.

18 - Tips to Keep a Skinny Body

Start your day with a smooth food. Gently prepare your new pouch with the new day ahead with yogurt and fruit smoothies. Fruits contain 80% water so digestion is easy for your stomach. Include protein powder in your shake for your daily protein requirements.

Include easy-to-prepare egg dishes for additional protein requirements. An egg is packed with protein, low sodium content and various vitamins and minerals. You can fry it in olive oil, poach it or boil it.

You can scramble it and add veggies for a morning omelet. You can use non-fat butter to make it tasty for many people who had undergone gastric bypass cannot tolerate eggs. Furthermore, it is so easy to prepare.

You can also begin your day with whole grains but dilute it with water while cooking. Whole grains have a tendency to expand when eaten. Since your pouch is smaller, you might experience extreme fullness that may lead to vomiting.

Cook lunch and dinner using one-dish principle. This means looking for a recipe that contains all the macronutrients that you need. For example, a recipe of chicken enchilada contains protein, calcium, carbohydrates and other essential nutrients.

Chicken contains protein. If you include cheese in cooking, you get your calcium requirement for the day. The enchilada sauce contains vitamins and minerals because of the tomato ingredients.

Toss in your favorite salad ingredients for a hearty afternoon snack. Just remember to choose low-fat mayonnaise or dressing to minimize consuming fatty foods. Alternately, use lemon, a tablespoon of olive oil and a dash of salt and pepper for a simple salad dressing.

The Order of Eating Your Food

You have to follow a strict code of eating healthy to maintain your weight and to minimize risks of dumping syndrome. Even if it means repeating a set of a meal for the next month or so, you will have to follow a strict diet of nutritious food. You will have to take supplements and eat your food in a particular order for the rest of your life.

In eating your food, you eat the protein first. Protein is the most important nutrient. Even if you did not finish your meal, the important thing is you got your protein requirement first. Fifty percent of your daily nutrition requirement comes from eating protein food and taking protein supplements.

After eating your protein, eat the vegetables and fruits in your meal. These can be in the form of a smoothie, soup or solid cooked food. The last is the starchy food or grain. If you feel full after eating your veggies and fruits, you can stop eating. You do not need to eat everything on your plate.

Meditative Eating

Is there such a thing as meditative eating? Yes, there is. Meditative eating, in other words, mindful eating, is connecting with your body's signal for fullness and hunger. It is paying attention to your new stomach. Meditative eating lets you eat leisurely and be mindful of the serving portions of every meal. It helps you in achieving your goals and minimizing risks of nausea and dumping.

Meditative eating consists of five components. The first component is eating slowly. Give at least 20 minutes or more but not exceeding to 1 hour to finish one meal. Chew your food thoroughly.

The idea is to chew your food 20-30 times. Do not rush and put down your spoon and fork in between bites. The best time to practice mindful eating is when you are slightly hungry. Thus, eat on time. Schedule your mealtime and follow it strictly.

The second component is persistence. You will have to do meditative eating for the rest of your life. Doing it once or twice is not enough. Make it a habit. Before you know it, you are doing meditative eating automatically.

The third component is openness. Become aware of what is going on with your body, particularly with your stomach. Sometimes, meditative eating can be a relaxing endeavor. Sometimes, you feel agitated especially if you feel your stomach is not doing okay.

The fourth component is to forget all criticisms from other people. These criticisms create negative feelings. Morbidly obese people, like you, are prone to judgmental comments from other people who can never understand how you feel. Most of the times, when you eat a meal, you would think if the food you are eating will not gain you a pound or will the food you eat will help you lose weight.

Stop these thoughts. Start thinking that eating is part of your success in losing the weight you hated since you hit that 40 BMI. Eating is a nutritious habit that will help you in losing more weight because you need to sustain your body's need.

The last component is doing one thing at a time. If you are eating, concentrate on eating. Do not watch TV or read a book while eating. It's okay to listen to classical music or your favorite sounds while eating. Listening to a relaxing music may even help you enjoy your food and chew slowly.

After the surgery, you will face big changes, including on how you view food. With meditative eating, you can handle these changes without being overwhelmed. Use your inner and outer wisdom to practice meditative eating and experience a positive impact on the gastric bypass operation in your life.

Outer wisdom refers to your basic knowledge of gastric bypass, to professional help from your surgeon and dietitian and experiences of other people with the same situation as you are.

Reading a book similar to this is also considered as an outer wisdom. Inner wisdom is your connection with your basal needs, your hunger and fullness signals and your stomach's reaction to the food you eat and drink. This also includes the feelings you experience before and after eating, emotionally and physically.

Aside from wisdom, it is important to appreciate the quality of the food you eat, instead of quantity. This is another aspect of meditative eating that you should practice. Perhaps, your parents have ingrained in your mind that everything you place on your plate should go to your stomach.

No food should be wasted. While this is the right thing to do, with your current state of a smaller stomach, you do not need to eat everything. To avoid wasting food, eat your meal one at a time. Just remember to eat the protein first before eating the vegetables and fruits. If you cannot really finish what you have prepared, freeze the remaining food and eat it for your next meal.

As you practice meditative eating, you will get a better understanding of how your stomach works. You will be able to estimate the amount of food you can eat in one sitting. Quality is the amount of nutrition you can get from a meal despite its smaller portion size. It refers to the freshness of the food, not processed or frozen to keep its shelf life.

Take Note of Portion Sizes

While eating slowly can contribute to losing weight and keeping your body free from complications, you should also be mindful of the serving sizes of your meals. It is useless to eat slowly and chew your food thoroughly if you are eating more than the recommended portion sizes for your new stomach.

Make it a habit of measuring and weighing the food you eat. Over time, you feel confident how a ½ cup of cereal or grains will look like in a bowl. There is nothing wrong if you know you can measure your food without needing a weighing scale. From time to time, check your measurements with the weighing scale and measuring cups and spoons.

However, there will be times that measuring becomes impractical, especially if you dine out occasionally or eat at a party. It is best to know a few guidelines in measuring portion sizes without actually using any measuring tool.

Drinking the Right Way

Water is an essential part of your post bariatric surgery. It helps your body distribute the necessary nutrients derived from the food you eat. Water keeps you hydrated, making your body function at an optimum level. Despite its importance, drinking the right way after the surgery is important.

Stop drinking at least 30 minutes before any meal. This will give your stomach enough time to do its work of distributing the water to your body parts. Resume drinking water at least 30 minutes after a meal.

Avoid drinking water and eating a meal at the same time. Water will push your food immediately to your intestines, making you eat more than usual. The worst thing is experiencing dumping syndrome.

There should be no alcohol during the first 10 weeks of recovery. Your new pouch is swollen and healing during these weeks. If you can manage, remove drinking alcohol altogether. Too much alcohol in your diet will not be good for your new stomach.

Avoid drinks with more than 10 grams of sugar. Many persons who had bariatric surgery notice that they suffer vomiting and dumping when they consume drinks with more than the 10-gram mark. Use natural sweeteners such as honey. You can use a sugar substitute to sweeten your drinks but use it sparingly. If you are bored with plain water, you can always spice up your drink with ginger, lemon or mint.

Sip your drinks. Do not gulp. Your stomach might rebel. Drinking in one gulp may cause vomiting. The worst thing is gulping may stretch your stomach. Gulping on a regular basis will hurt your stomach and may cause the staple and incision to open.

Drink the recommended water intake every day. During the first few weeks, your water intake may be limited to 1 liter a day. Every week, increase your water intake until you reach 2 liters a day.

Eating out, a possibility or not?

There would be times that you cannot help but eat out, either at a restaurant or at a get-together party or gathering. Gastric bypass surgery might have brought drastic changes in your life but it does not mean you give up all the things you enjoy before the surgery.

You cannot decline a date out with your loved ones, all the time. From time to time, you can still indulge in the pleasure of dining out. Your surgeon can even give you an identification card indicating you have undergone a gastric bypass surgery and that you need smaller serving sizes and healthier food servings that the restaurant is serving.

The employees of the restaurant can make changes for you. Some may ignore your request. Fortunately, more restaurants now are serving nutritious foods.

Surviving in a restaurant or fast food should not be a nightmare. Remember these tips and you can survive eating at a restaurant or fast food without experiencing any of the complication. Do not order food that indicates deep-frying or has a creamy sauce or crispy filling as part of the description. Most likely, these foods are high in fats. When dining out, you can request to place your salad dressing on the side.

Opt for veggie alternatives instead of an all-meat menu. For pizza restaurants, order a pizza with thin crust and more vegetables. Skip the pepperoni and sausages. For pasta menus, ask for the whole wheat variety with red sauce, instead of creamy white sauce.

In burger joints, you can order grilled patties instead of fried. When dining out in an Asian restaurant, order steamed veggies and meat. Skip fried rice. Instead, request for brown rice. Use chopsticks to slow you down when eating.

Keeping a Food Journal

During the weeks of your recovery and even after recovering and achieving your ideal weight, keep a food journal. A food journal is your lifelong tool in maintaining your weight. You should not stop writing in your journal. According to research, people who maintain a food journal lose more weight than those who do not keep one.

Jotting down everything you eat, a number of calories consumed can help you track down if you are eating right. This food journal can boost your confidence. It can improve your understanding of the reason you are eating.

Writing down your emotions and your cravings can help you evaluate what you really feel. It can help you think of alternate ways to divert your attention away from these cravings.

During the time when you are trying to achieve your weight loss goals after the surgery, cravings will become normal occurrences. Writing these cravings down in your journal will help assess your true feelings and what situations bring such cravings.

A food journal can help you plan your daily meals. You can write down your plan early in the morning as you sip your first no-sugar coffee or low-fat milk of the day. Planning what you will eat during the day is one-step away from your success. If you write down all symptoms and complications after eating a certain meal, you can identify specific patterns on how your stomach reacts to food.

Your food journal is not only for your own benefit. Your surgeon and dietitian can review your food journal to see how you are doing, especially if the supposed results of losing optimal weight are not favorable.

You can create a template for your food journal, which you can fill up as the day progresses. On the heading part, you can place the time of the day such as breakfast, lunch, dinner, morning snack or afternoon snack. You can also include the specific time of the day.

You can format it in a table form wherein the first column contains your meal plans and the corresponding measurements for each food to eat and liquid to drink. You should include the supplements you are taking or any exercise regimen you are following.

On the second column, write the remarks or any effect of the food or liquid you have consumed. These remarks may include any nauseous or vomiting episodes, stomach pain or cramping. Other information should include calorie intake, protein, and ounces of liquid consumed.

Alternatively, you can use an online food journal to keep track of your food consumption. Install this on your smartphone or laptop.

19 - Conclusion

Your responsibilities include making the right decisions when it comes to the food you eat, staying healthy and managing health complications while you recover. Keep your kitchen organized so you can eat healthily. Learn the different ways to cook and prepare healthy and nutritious foods. Manage health complications after the surgery. Achieve your goals and be healthy for the rest of your life.

Again, this is a long-term commitment. Along the way, you might commit mistakes in choosing the food to eat, the liquid to drink or the alternatives to the food ingredients you cook. Make your mistakes as learning opportunities to become more cautious. Your journals will aid you in improving your healthy lifestyle.

The final word is experimenting and exploring different healthy recipes is the key to variety and healthy eating. Actually, you can eat anything as long as it is in smaller portion sizes and at a reduced amount of fats. As long as you eat slowly and drink plenty of liquids, you are doing fine. Lastly, always have a follow-up check-up with your doctors. They know what to do when you are uncertain of everything.

Thank You

As we reach the end of this book, I want to say thanks for reading this book.

I want to get this information out to as many people as possible. If you found this book helpful, I would greatly appreciate you leaving me a review. This helps others find the book as well.

This book was self-published with the amazing help of <u>Self-Publishing Made Easy Now!</u> [3] . You can grab a free copy of the checklist that started my journey here: <u>FREE Self-Publishing Checklist</u> [4] .

[3]https://selfpublishingmadeeasynow.com/xpjv
[4]https://selfpublishingmadeeasynow.com/free_checklist

Disclaimer

This document is geared towards providing exact and reliable information in regards to the topic and issue covered. The publication is sold on the idea that the publisher is not required to render an accounting, officially permitted, or otherwise, qualified services. If advice is necessary, legal, financial, medical or professional, a practiced individual in the profession should be ordered.

This information is not presented by a financial or medical practitioner and is for entertainment, educational and informational purposes only. The content is not intended as a substitute for professional medical advice, diagnosis, or treatment. Always seek the advice of your physician or other qualified health care provider with any questions you may have regarding a medical condition. Never disregard professional medical advice or delay in seeking it because of something you have read.

The information provided herein is stated to be truthful and consistent, in that any liability, in terms of inattention or otherwise, by any usage or abuse of any policies, processes, or directions contained within is the solitary and utter responsibility of the recipient reader. Under no circumstances

DISCLAIMER

will any legal responsibility or blame be held against the publisher for any reparation, damages, or monetary loss due to the information herein, either directly or indirectly.